THE HEAL[ING GOSPEL]
OF SAINT JOHN

Essene Therapeutics by the Gnostic Founder of Christianity - THE NEW COMPLETE VERSION By The Founder of The Vitalogical Sciences
J. LOVEWISDOM, N.H.D., M.D., Sc.D, Ps.D, Ph.D, D.D.

POPULARIZED BY A 1/8th PORTION OF PROF. EDMOND BORDEAUX SZEKELY'S VERSION OF A SIMILAR VATICAN CODEX PUBLISHED IN 1939. "Essene" or "Therapeutic" means the HEALING or Healer's, as well as being the translation of "Jesus" or "Savior", which are all titles or names given to Saint John. GOD SPELL is the original English translation of "God Entrancement" or God-Rapture now spelled "Gospel", hiding the Esoteric Significance, in Christ Consciousness. Perfect Christians are the Gnostics or Saints, while Johanan means the God-Endowed, or Grace of God, referring to the Christ, or Anointed with the Holy Spirit, Gnosis. Our Complete uncensored new English translation of the full John Scroll from a Samaritan original, reveals the true original Spirit of The GNOSTIC FIRST CHRISTIANS OF ST. JOHN,- rejecting the tyranny of both Rome's politics and Jewish Slaughterhouse-Temple worshipers and scriptural doctrines. After the fall of Jerusalem, the great heroes among Essenes became the monastic ideal of Carmelite tradition, but in a Roman Church supporting Roman dogmatism and Imperialism. The Essene Spirit,- rooted in their Buddhist missionary origins from India,- with beliefs in a rigid Vegetarianism, Reincarnation, etc.,- were banned by Roman Church Councils, along with Gnostic tenets, holding to the Buddhist, Yoga and Universal Spiritual Oneness, in moral essentials, but with Freedom in theological and metaphysical theories. St. John, the Baptist,- or the 'Spiritually Anointed Savior Exalted' (the Aramaic meaning of Jesus Christ Crucified) with his Disciples,- gave rise to the allegories and wonders in HEALING told of in the Biblic legends, as amply explained in our text. The Gnostic Apostles of John were responsible for writing the N.T. Bible, as we reveal, and thus, a wholly new concept of Primitive Christianity, as it really was, unveils, also vindicated by Gnostic Scrolls. Our illustrations represent an ancient pictographic Paradisian origin of the Cross (+) as a Symbol for Immortal Divine Spirit, and the Tree of Life;- the Symbol of Aramaic: "Crucified" at Sunrise, O in X used by the Essene Order of Mt. Carmel as their symbol, and at Antioch, the Greek letter "X" (or Christ), was adopted in naming the Christened, Anointed, with Crucifixion-allegory of John's preaching, baptizing, life, and resurrection. "Wise as Serpents, harmless as doves", in the Spirit of Essenes, Gnostics evolved a "Mystical Body of Christ" in the N.T. Bible. Only Mother Nature and her Angels heal. Secrets told in this new Complete Scripture.

Edited and Translated by
DR. JOHNNY LOVEWISDOM

The Healing God Spell Of Saint John
San Francisco California USA
www.paradisianpublications.com

Disclaimer notice: This book is sold for information purposes only and is not intended as medical advice. The information in this book does not diagnose, prescribe, treat or cure any diseases, rather it promotes general health and well-being through better nutrition, exercise and lifestyle adjustments. The information given here is designed to help you make informed decisions about your health. It is not intended as a substitute for any treatment that may have been prescribed by your doctor. If you suspect that you have a medical problem, we urge you to seek competent medical help. The dietary programs in this book are not intended as a substitute for any dietary regimen that may have been prescribed by your doctor. As with all diet programs you should get your doctor's approval before beginning. All forms of diets and lifestyle changes pose some inherent risk, therefore the editors and publisher advise readers to take full responsibility for their safety and know their limits. Due to the fact that there is always some risk involved, the author, publisher and distributors of this book are not responsible for any adverse effects or consequences resulting from the use of any suggestions or procedures described herein. Neither the author, the publisher, nor the distributors will be held accountable for the use or misuse of the information contained in this book.

Copyright © 2009 All Rights Reserved
Reproduction or translation of any part of this work by any means, electronic or mechanical, including photocopying, beyond that permitted by the Copyright Law, without the permission of the publisher, is unlawful.

Printed in the United States of America

ISBN-13 978-0-9725877-4-7
ISBN-10 0-9725877-4-8

Diploma
Sacrorum Studiorum Collegium Academicum
Apud Sheffieldensem Urbem in Brittania Maion
(The Ministerial Training College)

Omnis Hominibus Bonnae Voluntatis Obique
Terrarum Sedentibus.
Nos Examinatorum Consensus Collegii Academici
Sacrorum Studiorum.
Potestate atque facultatibus nobis gentium pactis communicatas.
cum diligentec perspecti smus studiorum curriculum nostrae, Filectissimae oe doctissimae
Joannes Amadus Apostolus Christi Lovewisdom
Patriarchus Archiepiscopus Ecuadori
Deterimus coa Academicum Ordinem ae renuntiamus cumeans
Doctorum
Sacrae Theologiae
Haer testamur, omnibus palam facimus et diploma hoc
dimittimus ad omnin idoneum
Manu nostra datum atque sigillomunitum die XXVII
mensis........Maius.............anno Domini MCMLXXII.....

Rector Magnificus

Actorum Custos.   *Facultatis Praeses.*
               Tabularum

THE NORTHERN PONTIFICAL ACADEMY
Chartered by the Syrian Orthodox Patriarch of Antioch
for the advancement of learning, and the Eglise Gnostique Chretienne, tradition gnostique chretienne alexandrine et johannite, Nantes en France

This is to Certify
That we, the Council, acting upon the authority granted to us and having examined the credentials and qualifications of
the
Dr. Johnny Lovewisdom
Ecuador
and who has given Satisfactory evidence of good
moral Character and Social Welfare we have conferred on the
above mentioned the Distinction of
Doctor of Sacred Theology (S. T. D.)
Honoris Causa
Together with all the Rights and Privilege pertaining thereto
AS PATRIARCH ARCHBISHOP OF ECUADOR
In testimony whereof we have issued this
diploma duly signed and sealed by the Hand of the President
this 30th day of November Nineteen Hundred Sixty-Eight

John Trsuna,
President
THE NORTHERN PONTIFICAL ACADEMY
OFFICIAL STAMP OF THE PRESIDENT

(Seal of the Archbishop of Denmark, Scandinavian Countries and Baltic States Incorporated in Denmark.) The above authorization also covers the CATHOLIC APOSTOLIC PRIMITIVE ANTIOCH ORTHODOX CHURCH
in its Charter, and thus Honoris Causa The Gnostic-Essene and "Heavenly Ecclesia of the Living God in Aeonion Revivification" (Heavenly Church of God) whose foundation this document commemorates, authorizing Dr. Johnny Lovewisdom as the Head of the Heavenly Hierarchy. Registered in Archives No. 42.

The Healing God Spell of Saint John

With Emanations of Love - Wisdom to unfold Immortal Divine Spirit within, like a fragrant blossoming Rose, may you too hearten unto Cosmic Insight of a Living Oneness of our True - Being! THE HEALING GOD SPELL OF SAINT JOHN FINALLY - THE COMPLETE ARAMAIC ORIGINAL OF **The Essene Gospel of John** PATRIARCH ARCHBISHOP OF THE GNOSTIC CHRISTIANS OF SAINT JOHN and Apostolic Primitive Antioch Orthodox Catholic Church since 1968, the Essene Order of Mt. Carmel (The White Friars) since 1959, and Founder of the Paradisians. THE PRISTINE ORDER OF PARADISIAN PERFECTION The Most Sublime and Strictest Discipline on Earth ALSO KNOWN AS THE AUGUST ORDER OF LIVING IMMORTALS **THE HEALING GOD SPELL OF SAINT JOHN TRANSLATED AND EDITED FROM ARAMAIC BY DR. JOHNNY LOVEWISDOM, APOSTLE BELOVED OF CHRIST, PATRIARCH ARCHBISHOP OF THE HEAVENLY ECCLESIA OF THE LIVING GOD, Apostolic Successor of the Gnostic First Christians of Antioch, Syrian Orthodox Apostolic Church of Johanine and Alexandrian Tradition (1968), Reunited with the Apostolic Catholic Church (1972). With Emanations of LOVE-WISDOM To ALL! The NEW AGE MESSAGE. + The cross is a symbol for Divine Immortal Spirit** Dr. Lovewisdom was vested with the Habit (Garment) of the Essene Order of Mount Carmel, known as the "WHITE FRIARS" or Carmelites in the Strictest Tertiary Order on May 14th 1959 in Quito and given the Religious Name of "John of the Cross" ((the "+" or Cross) or Yoke (Yoga) is used by those who are Christed (the + pr. X is the Greek letter called "Christ") which also means Anointed with the IMMORTAL DIVINE SPIRIT, the Gnosis). Prior to that, he had also been ordained with a Minister's License, with his Doctorate as a Metaphysician or Spiritual Healing Practitioner by THE BROTHERHOOD OF THE WHITE LODGE, Inc. in the U.S.A. in 1949, after his Initiation as the Tashi Hutulktu, Kut Humi Lal Singh, successor to Pr. Dr. O.M. Chenrezi Lind, of THE GREAT WHITE BROTHERHOOD, LODGE AND LOTUS ORDER OF GURUS of Tashi Lumpo, Shigatse, Tibet and Tiwa, Sin Kiang in 1948 as the Maha Chohan of the 7th Root Race, and the Living Buddha Maitreya, beside already being recognized as the Father of the New Race and the New Age since 1942, the Reincarnation of John the Illumined (or Baptist) in 1944. Copyright 1978 by ++ Dr. Johnny Lovewisdom. All Rights Reserved. Copies Available for $10.00 Bank Check, airmailed. +++ (From the 1978 printing) Published (Publicado por) by LA PRENSA DE UNIVERSIDAD INTERNATIONAL, Casilla H, Loja, Ecuador. (Address no longer valid) HIS HYPERBOREAN HOLINESS. THE HEAD OF THE HIGHER HEAVENLY HIERARCHY CENOBIO "EL PARAISO" Publicado por la Prensa de UNIVERSIDAD INTERNACIONAL FUENTE DE CIENCIAS VITALOGICAS CELESTE ECCLESIA DEL DIOS VIVO, Orden Pristina de la Perfeccion Paradisiaca, Reg. Of. 892 Acdo. 1725-18-IX-75 del Ecuador, Casilla H, Loja, Ecuador THE RESURRECTION SEAL OF LOVEWISDOM: John, Apostle Beloved of Christ, Patriarch Archbishop of the Seven Churches of Asia, embracing Catholic, Orthodox, All Eastern and Gnostic First Christians, Essene, Therapeutae, Parsee, Sufi, Taoist, and Yoga tenets; Buddhist Tashi Hutulktu Jnana Karuna, Maitreya Buddha Incarnate: Oneness of ALL, THE HEAVENLY ECCLESIA of Living God Divinely Directed by The PRISTINE ORDER OF THE PARADISIAN PERFECTION, in the Strictest Discipline on earth. To realize the strict abstinence from the Active Causative Substances that give origin to Cravings, Lust and Disease, as the Basic Source of Thoughts, Attachment and a Life in Sin:- WE FORSAKE the consuming of eggs, nuts, grains, legumes and other SEEDS, - which augment Reproductive Substance-Activities; beside fish, fowl or all animal FLESH, cooked foods, leather, pesticides, drugs, etc., - which augment Killing or destroy Sentient Life. The ideal of this Spiritualizing Dietetics, or VITARIANISM, is eating only Juicy Fruit, - supplemented with succulent vegetables, when necessary. When one achieves true Sublimation of Libido thus, thru our precise Dietetic Science of Continence, or VITALOGY, one eliminates and heals menstruation as well as seminal losses. Only while this Natural Reproductive Control does exist, - do we allow the use of 10 to 20 % avocados or clabber (a bacterial plant culture) to dress Raw Vegetable Salads. All Sin and Unhappiness is the Lack of Love for our Creator and for one another. When we live by loving, also as male and female, one in the Image of God, sustained by Living Water in juicy fruits of Paradise,- the ideal we live for,- we shall be Perpetually Born again from our embryonic seed if we retain it within and nourish this Agape of Love. Thus, we Forsake the World of Sin, Crime, Deception and its evil Karma to **BUILD PARADISES** to be with God and to Nourish from the **JUICY FRUITS,- HIS HEALING, SAVING AND LIVING WATER OF LIFE EVERLASTING!** // **ONLY THRU THE PRACTICE OF THIS PARADISIAN LIFE OF IMMACULATE CONCEPTION, WITHOUT BLOODSHED, POPULATION EXCESSES, WAR AND CONSEQUENT ECOLOGIC PLAGUES, - CAN THE NEW AGE AND RACE SURVIVE!**

FOREWORD:-
HOW TO BE SAVED AND GAIN THE UNATTACHED LOVE-WISDOM FACTOR

Before all the scattered vignettes, oracles or "Sayings of the Savior" occurring unorderly like the "Gnostic Gospel of St. Thomas, were assembled into a narrative to tell the Story of Christna, but fulfilling the Old Testament prophecies, in what is now known as the NEW TESTAMENT, the private life of John (meaning God-Endowed in Aramaic, hence Savior, Anointed by the Holy or Christ Spirit) was much different than the "all things to all people" scriptural accommodations invented to fit into a theory of Immaculate Conception preached about all Saviors. The Great White Brotherhood, Lodge (Ekklesia) and Order of Essenes, with Sanctuary-Colleges in the foothills of Mt. Carmel (White Friars), like their Eastern Brethren in the Lamaseries of Tibet and the Himalayas (with their "Bhagavad-Gita", "Songs of Milarepa", etc.), wove deep allegorical narratives that capture the reader's mind to illustrate cosmic principles of Spiritual Truth. Often, only small fragments of recognizable historic fact remain decorated by artistic literary Spiritual Conceptions of heart-begotten Love and mind-born Wisdom narrated, except to those who can witness the Living Word in a New Spiritual Birth within.

John tells of his former life before he had "risen from the dead", as the Anointed Savior (Jesus Christ), or "born again of Holy Spirit and Living Water", saying: "Among those born of women, there is not a greater prophet than John, the Illumined" (Baptist is mistranslation, Lk. 7:28). After the Feb. 16, 1542 Convocation of Papal Bishops, 99 "Sacred Words" were revised in the N.T. Bible to hide their original meaning, occurring with Protestant versions also, altho the first English N.T. of Wycliffe in 1360, translated from Old "Vetus Italica" of the second century, used "Healer" or "Healing man" in place of Jesus or Savior, and "God-Spell" or God Entrancement instead of Gospel. Baptism roots in dawn, sunrise or day light meaning Illumination, John being Illumined, Initiator or Founder of Christianity which Roman papists wanted to hide, crediting "Peter"

The Illumination (Baptism) occurred on the Jordan at BETHANY, which means "House of Figs", but fig trees have gum "tears", leaves wail or moan in wind; beside echo, which allegorically led to Tearful Mary, repenting sins. It was at the crossing, thus christening (+) of Jordan, still another meaning, that the Savior was Anointed with the Holy Spirit thru Mary's Love at Bethany, and John was born again of the Holy Spirit by Immaculate Conception. Simon was not a "leper" his house being of pots or a potter's house, Simon meaning Listener, so dwelling pots, or the container of soul meant body-conscious. John translates to mean "God-Endowed", he is son of "Zebedee" (meaning God, the Endower) as well as "Zachary" (also meaning God-penetration, or born of Spiritual Consciousness). Zachary's house was at "Bethlehem", meaning House of Bread, Sustenance or Living. There are thus 2 Bethanys, 2 Bethlehems, 2 Johns, 2 James, 2 Marys, etc. giving Gnostic allegories as to body and spiritual consciousness, flesh and Spirit, but the political Papacy hid all this by adding genealogies and other data making "Jesus" a historical man, replacing John, the origin.

Historically, Josephus records that he was also a follower of BANUS, but Banim means sons, like "Sons of Prophets" as Essenes of Mt. Carmel were called (2 Kings 6:1) initiated "Sons of God", so Banus may have been John or Jesus (Savior), the key originals being censored or lost. That John wore camel hair and skin is unthinkable, the Aramaic word meaning rope beside camel, so he wore rope hemp garment, which grow wild, just as he ate what grew of itself, referring to Carob husks or fruit, not locusts, being of the locust bean tree. John ate no bread, drank no wine and killed not.

The National Cancer Institute just announced research findings that boiling food caused mutations in protein, giving cancer causing factor, so with earlier warning against carcinogenic hydrocarbons resulting from broiling and roasting, all cooked or "dead" food is being scientifically proven disease-producing as John historically taught, as well as "Jesus" who gave the key to "Fount of Living Water Springing up into Life Everlasting" as Living Food (Bread) for born again Spirit and true Sons of God. Excess Phosphorous, in the seed substances as food, super phosphate fertilizer, Organophosphate pesticides, etc. displace calcium the king-pin of mineral-balance in the body, causing caries, and most other diseases.

"PROLOGUE" (as given by the Samaritan Order for) "THE HEALING GOD SPELL OF SAINT JOHN"

"Here within we present:
THE SECRET DOCTRINE that Christ taught in his time to a select group of Disciples, under the leadership of Saint John, in order that this teaching might be published and taught in our present time, and thus only being released at the start of the Twentieth Century. (1899) This Healing God Spell reveals the Secrets of the Way to acquire a long and pleasant life, enjoying therein the fullest use of the physical, mental and psychic faculties without pain or sickness, with a plenitude of material blessings, spiritual gifts, of an imperturbable peace and the ineffable joy of living in everlasting contentment. 'AGAIN, I HAVE MANY OTHER THINGS TO TELL YOU, BUT YOU CANNOT GRASP THEM NOW' (St. John 16:12).

With these words the Christ meant that there remained much wisdom to be revealed, but the time had not come to teach all of this because mankind was not ready to receive such advanced knowledge. This is the reason why Christ did not publicly teach all his doctrine, except to a privileged few, in secret, a chosen group of disciples led by Saint John, so that when the time was ripe this doctrine would be publicly taught."

This is how the thus named HEALING GOD SPELL OF SAINT JOHN was born which this illustrious Disciple condensed into 42 Chapters, whose original was carefully guarded thru-out time by the millennial Samaritan Order, founded by the Divine Master at the time he issued forth the precious parable of the Good Samaritan.

Thus, we publish the English translation of the Aramaic original that was conserved at the famous University LIBRARY OF ALEXANDRIA, arduous protector of Greek, Egyptian and all ancient Arts and Letters, of which various translations exist, including Spanish (among those we carefully compared ours with).

The mentioned Library containing the most valuable works from most ancient times of inestimable value, was burned by uncontrollable hordes of the invading armies, but we have obtained our translation from the original God Spell manuscript miraculously saved because this papyrus original had been carefully protected in fired clay jars hidden in secret vaults.

Altho this Healing God-Spell (Gospel) has appeared in various apocryphal editions, in mutilated, partial and incomplete forms, issued from the hands of various translators who were cautiously only given parts of the originals and never the complete text for their translations, the present version is published as truthfully as it was transmitted. THIS IS THE FULL, COMPLETE AND AUTHENTIC ENGLISH VERSION PUBLISHED FOR THE FIRST TIME.

"This is because the very Spirit of Christ watches over these precious originals, due to the doctrine they contain, having such an exalted destiny to accomplish in future cultural advancements, for which it was specially designed. Already at that time it was known that in the 20th Century was precisely the time for publishing this teaching (see Apoc. 20:4-6), when mankind would be prepared to understand, assimilate and, above all, realize its practice in everyday living. Up to that time, the study of the Holy Bible was enough preparation and has made it known that Christ is comparable to a grain of wheat which if not planted remains inert, but as soon as it is planted, it issues forth an abundant harvest of grain identical to the one originally planted.

This verse clarifies and makes reasonably understandable the MYSTERY OF GOLGATHA (in the Place of the Skull), the occult justification as to why Christ, notwithstanding his Omnipotent Powers, did not want to use them to free himself from his executioners, but freely submitted of his own will to being captured, insulted, spit upon, whipped, crowned with thorns, and finally crucified and buried in the earth. Thus, it was so his Spirit would become buried deeply in all human hearts and from there germinate, like a grain of wheat germinates in the earth, to ripen and finally in one immense human wheat field, give forth a fabulous harvest of CHRISTIANS, equal and identical in Divinity, Power, Harmony and Love to the original seed planted.

This is because each human being is in reality a CHRIST IN POTENTIALITY, in that, with the passing of time surely one will become so, complying with the Will of the SUPREME CREATOR.

Just as in schools, with each new period, new textbooks for more advanced studies are required, so are new teachings in Sacred Scriptures. Foreseeing all conditions in Life, the Divinity also foresaw preparation of Textbooks for Living to teach us. So in the propitious time the text of the most Sacred Scripture, the

Holy Bible, was prepared as the PRIMARY mystical, moral and religious Teaching, which thus in our present time has been fulfilled with the times we are living in, that is in this Age of Materialism, and differs with the SPIRITUAL NEW AGE. Just as the teachings of religions is realized in CYCLES, each of Two Thousand years duration, the First Cycle will be finished with the end of the present century, beginning a New Cycle, the foretold Spiritual Cycle.

For the Teaching of this New Age, the Divinity has foreseen a more intensive and penetrating study of the Holy Bible, and also to complement this wonderful Scripture, has prepared the foretold HEALING GOD SPELL OF SAINT JOHN. The great variety of teachings that this work contains, little by little shall elevate the culture and wisdom of the people, making them more brotherly, more noble, and of a more cosmic scientific advancement. This Cycle of Life shall be so advanced, so different and superior to the actual one, that all mankind shall be removed from its very foundations to give birth to it.

Then shall the SPIRIT RULE OVER MATTER, firmly holding the bridle reins of the body and leading it on the pleasant paths of Natural Living, confident in their purpose in human beings of the greatest enjoyment of Physical and Spiritual Health, awakening and revealing within them their highest abilities.

The only possibility of achieving this Sublime objective would be thru intensive training in INTEGRATED NATURAL LIVING which shall then become the OFFICIAL STATE TEACHING, taught from PRIMARY SCHOOLS TO THE UNIVERSITIES.

This Second Cycle will also only last two thousand years which shall be followed by a Third Cycle, when the Teaching shall include the astral and the heavenly planes, which, at the present time, remain beyond our understanding.

Fulfilling the aforementioned ideals of the SAMARITAN ORDER, we are pleased to make public the contents of the COMPLETE ORIGINAL MANUSCRIPT IN ARAMAIC. We have the devoted desire that this sublime doctrine descending from heaven, will adjust health teachings to all social levels, to bring them up to the Dawn-lit Peaks, of PURE TRUTH by the harmonious paths designed by our loving MOTHER NATURE. These are the only paths capable of leading us to the COMPLETE REGENERATION OF THE HUMAN SPECIES, by exterminating its vices and bad habits, moral and physical suffering and related evils, precisely caused by mankind's neglect or ignorance of the Transcendental Truth and Teachings of the Divine Masters.

Our Guiding Angel would love to guide the footsteps of those who are eager to find the Healing Fountain of Regeneration, to give us a hand to support our efforts to reach these Dawn-lit Peaks, where the SUN OF TRUTH unfurls all its beneficial rays, without being eclipsed by the dense mists of Ignorance, Prejudice, Errors and Vanities that cover it today.

THE INTERNATIONAL SAMARITAN ORDER"
Editor's Note: The above Prologue appeared with the Spanish Edition, "Evangelio de Salud de San Juan", which we have adjusted in translation to propitiously fit our English rendition, to give the exact information and explanation as to how and why our original manuscript in Aramaic rescued from the Alexandrian Library by the Samaritan Order, does not contain copyist interpolations, nor the OMISSIONS REMOVING SEVEN-EIGHTHS OF THE ORIGINAL MANUSCRIPT which Prof. Dr. Edmond Bordeaux Szekely's translation of the Vatican Library Aramaic Codex contained. Usually, as explained in our "Introduction", the Roman Church or the Vatican has taken the originals that the public liked, and eliminated "the poison of false doctrines", contrary to their dogma, to return these Scriptures with omissions or interpolations for public use. Being of the Carmelite Order or Essenes or First Christians of Samaria, I well know how well Truth is thus censored within the Papal Catholics of Rome. It would have been hard to get a full Aramaic Vatican mss. copy in Prof. Szekely's time, hand-copying old papyrus, etc. even if repeated visits to do it were allowed. As to Prof. Szekely's story that archaeology was unable to reconstruct how the Nestorian priests got his Royal Hapsburg Library Slav version, it is especially strange.

Why this branch of Eastern Church Nestorians would value and rescue a Monophysite manuscript, or of their enemies, seems illogical. The story of Jesus transfiguring from a human body appearance, created by auto-hypnotic mystical experience or initiation, the God Spell of intensive faith and meditation, as known also in the Spiritual Nature of vivid dreams and clairvoyant visions or visits, into a heavenly figure levitation into radiant light like the moon or sun (Chapter XII Szekely version and Chapter XIII here within) illustrates the Monophysite,

5   The Healing God Spell of Saint John

Alexandrian Gnostic and Samarian First Christians of St. John doctrine. Nestorians hold that Jesus was a man of history. We received written permission from the International Samaritan Order Headquarters in Santiago, Chile for our English version, also of the Great White Brotherhood in the Andes. (The Editor's Notes, giving alternate meanings or clarification, are in PARENTHESES).

"GOOD SAMARITAN" GNOSTIC CHRISTIANS OF
SAINT JOHN THE BAPTIST

As the most ancient Order of Knightly Nobility, the INTERNATIONAL SAMARITAN ORDER seeks out Human Souls of Real Aristocracy and genuine moral beauty, showing faultless behavior in right living, a conduct free of vice and dedicated to Natural Living. The Order was established after the model of the Good Samaritan of the New Testament, in Selfless Service of true Brotherly Love and the Regeneration of Mankind by teaching each person to become their own healer and priest. The former international center in the USSR sector of Berlin (whose last honorary president was Empress Augusta Victoria of Germany) has been relocated in Santiago, Chile.

In a course of study in Spanish that the International Samaritan Order began to publish in 1944, "Plan Evolutivo del Mundo" (3 volumes), the authors state that this Plan is of the true Government of Governments, often described as the GREAT WHITE BROTHERHOOD of the Masters of Wisdom that have guided mankind for the last 18 million years from various hidden mt. retreats on earth.

With well-chosen brief illustrations, this text shows how in the New Spiritual Age mankind will consciously accept a government ruled by the Most Qualified, true Masters of Wisdom, rather than past monarchies, dictatorships and the popular vote of the ignorant masses, all of whom follow their sensual dictates rather than higher guidance in Love and Wisdom offered by the Masters, to give a faultless reform in education,- hygiene based on strict natural diet, living and healing, and the Union or Religion of all Faiths in One Religion of Love, all coming about by the spontaneous growth of man learning by painful experience from suffering ages of error. Man evolves thru error and pain that build the virtues that bless mankind with health, happiness and peace within.

This Plan of the Samaritan Order states: "The Famous GNOSTIC DOCTORS were the True Masters of Wisdom, whose inspiration became the Christian Religion (perverted in practice), and originated with the Wise Men who came from the Orient who were the only ones who knew when and where the Christ would appear to leave the Gnostic Gems and Treasures described in the N.T. Bible, actually being emissaries of the Great White Brotherhood. The Gnostics taught the Law of Karma (Cause and Effect), Reincarnation, and many truths Christians avoid.

In another work distributed by the Samaritans "Error de un Jesuita" (by Carlos Otero V.) it states quoting about the famous Gnostic Christian: "St. Clement of Alexandria (120-220) in his work 'Paidagogos' defended his position against the abominable practice of eating animal flesh saying: "Is it not true that within our frugal simplicity, there exists a great variety of healthy foods: greens, bulbs, olives, salads, fruits and so many other vegetarian food products? Among these foods we should give Preference to those we can eat in their natural state without the use of fire. Flesh foods paralyze the Spiritual Faculties. Thus, the Gnostics abstained from flesh foods seeking to avoid inclinations to lustful desires by their bodies. Such food is condemned."

St. Basil the Great, Church Father and Patriarch of Eastern Monastic Orders held: "The body is burdened by flesh foods, it becomes infected by disease and the decomposition of such abominable food darkens the Light of the Spirit. No matter what the animal flesh may be, all of them always give rise to impure actions. In terrestrial Paradise there was no wine or killing of animals, or flesh foods. As soon as we begin to live frugally and rationally Happiness will rule our homes, there will be no bloodshed and our tables will only have the fruits and vegetables of Nature giving growing satisfaction to all." St. John Chrysostom and other Eastern Church Fathers gave identical views.

From the aforementioned text of the Samaritans, I shall condense some more of the author's views: "What is the origin of the monstrous habit of killing and the shedding of animal blood in the worship of God? The religious teachers of the antiquity...taught that man's body, or the animal part should be subdued and sacrificed for the Spirit, to overcome vice and evil habits or deliver him from his sins. But in time this was taken to mean that the beast or animal flesh, that man domesticated outside his body, was to be sacrificed or killed for Spirit, to please God as practiced by the Jews. Moses received his education in Egypt, pampered by the king's daughter, unworthily taught the magical arts and Egyptian Mysteries, while he came to use them as black arts for killing, war, slaughtering Ethiopians, deception and other crimes.

But let us take a glimpse at the Temple and Doctrine which he laid foundations for in his teaching. Going within the Temple of Jerusalem one could witness the sacrifice of slaughtered beasts by innumerable priests, working in shifts, who killed the innocent animal victims, hung up the carcasses, disembowelled and burned their offal parts in an enormous holocaust, peeled off their skins and finally delivered each ritually consecrated carcass to their donors. Blood covered the floor up to the ankles of the priests, whose white robes became completely stained to the color of blood. Truly, never has a greater Slaughterhouse existed, and such an abominable monstrosity was dedicated to Jehovah (Yahweh) as a Temple. Watching only 6 hours, an estimated ten thousand victims were sacrificed, 256,000 in one Pasch. Belonging to the Altar, a gigantic oven 16 meters square and 7 high, fired constantly from below, was attended to by 70 priests who received the sacrificial victims like processing in a modern meat packing factory.

How could these Priests of the Old Law,- who produced so much pain and shed the blood of so many victims, have any true concept of God, Spirit, Love?

How could Moses have talked with God, like man with man, and mystified God's "chosen people" in such practices, living as a war criminal and all the deception and plundering he did? The explanation rests precisely in the fact that whatever good may be found in him, such as the Ten Commandments, "Mosaic Law" and other Concepts of Yahweh, are all to be found in the Ancient "BOOK OF THE DEAD", texts which date before Jewish history, studied by Moses in Egypt. Chapter 17 and especially Chapter 125 reveal word for word the origin of their Commandments, to be Egyptian Doctrines. Engaged in crime, the Jewish tribes had no culture, religion or land of their own, all being usurped from others."

From the above condensed text of explanation, beside the "Secret Doctrine" of Helen Blavatsky and numerous other Bible critics, all evidence shows the Jewish doctrine and history to be pure myth, the fictitious repetition of the legends they purloined from Mesopotamia, Egypt, Arabia and Palestine, along with the wealth of whoever they were able to plunder from; those they victimized.

To cover up this long history of bloody butchery of peaceful peoples and monstrous crimes they admittedly boast about in their Scriptures, the Old Testament Law Giver, Moses became the "Angel Messiah" of ancient legend, who went about with a "magic Wand" or staff, which he could make turn into a Serpent, or cause to bring suffering and death in plagues, fire and a voice in a bush, water from a rock, and in an endless bag of tricks of Magic, conjure up dew that became food to feed his people for 40 years, win their wars, etc. A ruthless butcher of helpless people, a war criminal who killed the captives and was wroth with officers when they had not killed women and children, he established Mosaic Law, "Kill every male among the little ones (beside all adults) and kill every woman that hath known man. But all the virgin girls keep alive for yourselves." (Num. 31:17) The Holy men of Yahweh had the job of fingering all the pretty young women to see if they were virgins to serve for immoral purposes, while all other human captives were slaughtered and their cities burned after plundering their riches. Their Bible established this Law.

Just as we have established the allegorical nature of New Testament facts in history, originally intended as symbolic tales and miracles wrought by a super-physical Spirit, "Jesus", that walks thru walls and locked doors etc. completely hiding the identity in the resurrect spirit of the beheaded Saint John the Baptist; to which the etherealized deeds in the Zealot rebellion to Jewish and Roman Government in Palestine were integrated, the Old Testament likewise was fabrications of Nazarite and Essene allegorical writers in the tradition of Egyptian Hierophants versed in the Mysteries. For this, from the earliest time, the tribe of Levi was made free of war and warring expeditions, their welfare being taken cared of as a gift from God, receiving tithes, which gratuity claimed that the Nazarites or Essenes should write flattering tales for historical record to be used to Model future generations. Crime and sin of the Jews were overlooked as being counselled by Yahweh. In the same way the religious orders and Saints of the Roman Church and Holy Empire became the soul, model or "front" for the Inquisition and the Conquistadores. All men tend to defend their homeland. Not to do so has meant death often.

Symbolically, the rod of Levi blossoming to bear fruit, revealed the Biblical Forbidden Food to be almonds, lacking Living Water and reproductive substance begetting a lusting reproductive nature to the consumer. Like the religious orders preaching of not killing, but harbouring self-righteousness for killing among their countrymen, the cultivation of peaches, apricots, etc. that are exploited for seed food (almonds, walnuts, etc.) become stumbling stones for those seeking the Living Water of Everlasting Life. This is why the Essenes, in spite of abstaining from killing and giving an "aura" of holiness to the Jewish nation, vanished from historical records after the fall of Jerusalem 70 A.D., taking away their hypocritical basis as Jews, henceforth being described among the Christian Gnostics. They loathed and repented their former collaboration perpetuating the Slaughterhouse Temple and plundering wars. Too often, religious ideals are exploited as tools or fronts for cover by sinners.

However, the mystical "Keys to the Kingdom of Heaven" that unlock the Mystery that reveals how Christianity owes its origins to the Gnostic First Christians of Saint John the Baptist, are to be found in the New Testament Bible itself. In John's Gospel we read: "There was a man sent from God whose name was John (which in Aramaic is written "God's Grace" or "Gift"). This man came as a witness to give testimony of the Light that all men might believe thru him...That was the true Light which enlighteneth every man that cometh into this world...John gave testimony saying, "I gaze upon the Spirit descending as a dove out of Heaven. It remained on him. Yet, I was not aware of Him but He Who sent me to baptize with water. (John saw no man, but the Spirit that led him to baptize.) That One said to me, "On WHOSOEVER you perceive the Spirit to descend and remain on him, this is He Who is baptizing in the Holy Spirit. I have seen and testified that this One is the Son of God. On the morrow JOHN AGAIN STOOD WITH TWO OF HIS OWN DISCIPLES and looking he saw the Savior ("Jesus") among them, and said "Behold the Lamb of God". (John has seen a lamb personifying the Savior, instead of the dove symbol just mentioned, showing he is speaking in ALLEGORIES like the Gnostics and Essenes).

And the two disciples followed this Savior. (In a like manner various Disciples witness the Spiritual Baptism of those in Christ meaning they were anointed with His Spirit, or Christened) ...From now on you will see Heaven opened and the angels (messengers) of God ascending and descending to the Son of mankind."

The first Chapter just quoted, speaks about the experience in the Gnosis. The testimony is of the Spirit among the Disciples of John. "What is born of flesh is flesh, and what is born of Spirit is Spirit...God is Spirit and they who worship Him must worship Him in Spirit and Truth". Those who worship man in the flesh, thus cannot be worshipping God who is Spirit and Truth. Jesus is the Son of God, or Spirit, and thus, He is the Spirit among His Apostles, not man with a self. In Chapter 4, it says "The Lord knew that Pharisees hear that the Savior is making and baptizing more disciples than John, though the Savior did not baptize, but His Disciples." Again, it shows the Light of the World was the Spirit that continued in the Disciples of John the Baptist (as the Gnostic Gospel writers claimed ever to be), and that they performed all their works of wonder in His Name, who did the works by the Father in Him. So the Disciples do the works He does, and even greater works than told of Him, Since the Father, Spirit and Truth does the works (Jn. 14:10, 12, 20).

When the Samaritan woman asked, the Savior Spirit in the Disciples answered, "If thou didst know John (the Grace or Gift of God), he would have...given you Living Water...He that drinks of the water that I will give him shall not thirst forever but that water shall become in him a fountain springing up into life aeonian...My food is to do the will of Him that sent me that I may make perfect his work." This food was told of in Genesis 1:29, where God gave herbs and fruits that yield up their seeds for planting, are to be our food, which is a 90% Living Water Diet. John "was a burning and shining Light" because his WORKS gave testimony of Jesus, and not that a man or self other than the Spirit and Truth that saves existed beside John and his Disciples. (See Jn. 5:33-36) "The Spirit will teach you, He will not speak of HIMSELF" (Jn. 16:13).

With the above Keys, the so-called historic or Synoptic Gospels are understood by showing the Savior (Jesus) to be the Spiritual Title that John was known by when seen continuing in the Disciples, who said the Savior travelled with them and did the works done in His Name by them. The Protevangelium, Book of James states that the Father of John Baptist, Zachary, knew the Virgin Mary in the Temple, when she was 14, altho she was raised by this priest and others since the age of 3 years. Mary conceived and lived in Zachary's home 3 months when the barren wife of Zachary in spiritual rapture felt "the Grace of God" (John) leaped into her womb. John was the Horn of Salvation come to give Knowledge of Salvation to his people, in other words, he was the Savior (Jesus) "the Orient from on High" thus (Luke 1:69, 77, 78). What is veiled in Scriptures authorized for the Bible is that John is the child of Zachary and Mary, who is presented as John the Baptist, giving the priestly office, but to avoid infant's slaughter, the stories of the Hidden Life of the Savior are told so as to give the Life of Jesus, the Name John taught as the doer of God's Word and Works among the Apostles. One can see why the Roman Church prohibited the translation and publication of Bibles, since it would reveal the Mystery of the Savior (Jesus) among the Gnostic Disciples of John the Baptist.

"The Kingdom of God is within you...For where 2 or 3 are gathered in my Name, there am I in midst of them"...The Word of God came to John...The people in their heart thought John was Christ...(they said Jesus or Savior) was John risen from the dead." The New Testament allegories reveal the Savior Spirit and Truth of John Baptist revivified in the Apostles, a Living God manifest as a Holy Spirit among men, altho their body form is not Spirit.

THE HEALING GOD SPELL OF ST. JOHN

The Original and Complete Aramaic Text now translated for the first time by the Apostle Beloved in Christ, Johnny Lovewisdom in Living Incarnation as the Patriarch Archbishop of the GNOSTIC FIRST CHRISTIANS OF ST. JOHN in combined Apostolic Authority from the Syriac Orthodox and Ancient Catholic Churches for the HEAVENLY ECCLESIA.

CHAPTER I (1-18)

In those days many that were sick and maimed came to the Saving Healing One, asking him, "Thou who knowest all things, tell us, why do we suffer these infirmities? Why do we suffer with illness and pain? Lord, heal us, that we too need not suffer, and that we may be of use to ourselves and to other humans. Thou who hast the power to heal us in thy hands, make us well and in good health again. Lord, free us from the power of Satan from whom we suffer. Master have compassion on us, do not forsake us and heal us."

The Anointed One answered: "Happy art ye who thirst and hunger for Wisdom, for I will satisfy thee with Living Water, that ye may never thirst (for other water) and I shall grant you knowledge of Living Bread (food) that ye may never hunger (for other bread). Blessed art ye who come to me filled with faith and knock at the only true Door to Knowledge and Wisdom that I may open it to you, wide without hindrance. Happy art ye who I shall free from Satan because I shall lead you into Mother Nature's Kingdom of Angels where only Joy and Happiness abide and from whose realm Satan is excluded.

John had always lived close to the Lord God, so that those who hungered for Wisdom, especially his own Elect Disciples, as well as many of their followers, listened attentively to his Divine Teaching lest any words of Wisdom escape unheard from this Divine Source, and occasionally asked their Teacher Anointed in the Spirit of Divine Wisdom (Gnosis, Christ) questions such as this: "Master, please explain to us, Who is our Mother Nature, and who are her Angels?

Thy Mother in Nature, or Creation, is within thee and you in her. She gave thee birth, thy body and all that you are because she gave you Life in Creation. And this body that she gave thee you must likewise each day return to thy Mother Nature. Happy art ye for you shall experience the unmeasurable Joy of knowing such a Good Mother and Her Kingdom. And ye shall know thy Holy Mother as soon as you receive Her Holy Angels devotedly, that is to say, as soon as you obey the Unchangeable Laws of Nature, because each Angel has one particular law to declare to you, one Divine Blessing to grant and one human virtue by which it is known. Now, let us embrace in Mind the Supreme Truth, that states: "Anyone whosoever strictly keeps the Commandments of our Mother in Nature, honoring them daily, SHALL NEVER BE SICK"! This is because the power of our Mother Nature is Infinite and Almighty thru-out Creation and full of the Creator's Infinite Wisdom, Love, Mercy and Beauty.

Mother Nature in her power of Great Compassion shall cast out Satan who takes possession of men's hearts, causing them to do evil, to defraud, to commit crimes and even to kill. Yet when Satan has been cast out of your heart, and it becomes the dwelling of the Angel of Life, your way of living will radically be changed: You shall become good, kind, righteous, honest and you shall love one another as much as yourself, including even those who hate you, and likewise, you shall love every creature that God created on earth. The Power of the Almighty within His Creation manifests thru-out Mother Nature, and thus, reigns in your body, and in the bodies of all living beings and even in the Mineral, Vegetable as well as Animal Realms.

//

Editorial Footnotes: Many people never really understood the Bible because it used the out-dated, anachronistic dialect of the 16th century, giving a dignified, mystical and forbidden aura as tho only the clergy could interpret such matters. To the other extreme, if the Aramaic N.T. Bible is stripped of all the multiple meanings of its words, we have only a small fraction of the Truth in the original significance. One Aramaic word is translated with up to 24 meanings. So, to establish the Spiritual Mood of Sacred Invocation seeking Truth, in this First Chapter we have used the solemn familiarity of "thee" and "thou" as found in "Our Father" and other prayers still in use. But henceforth we shall come forth in frank mid-twentieth-century language of greater scientific truth.

Yet, our plain-spoken revelation of Truth shall require great spiritual courage to accept: to some it will mean taking away what little they knew as to legendary biblical history and interpretation. Christians in general under Roman Church tutelage, including Protestants, have come to believe "Jesus Christ" was a man in the flesh separate from the Apostles, His Brethren and Sisters as well as Disciples, because the Key Words were never completely grasped or even translated completely. When the Jews asked John (who was called "Baptist", interpolated to match Josephus' writings), if he was the Anointed One (Messiah, Christus or Christ), he denied that God was manifest in his body, or to be seen as flesh. "No man has ever seen God but those first born of God, who are in the Father's bosom, as he (John) declared Him (God).

To clarify the meaning of the "Christ" or Anointed One, this must be first understood as anointing with Spirit, and not as ritual anointing with oil dependent on physical substances and persons. "The Spirit of the Lord is upon me, because the Lord has ANOINTED me and sent me to preach good tidings to the meek...You shall be named priests of the Lord and called ministers of God",- found in Isaiah 61:1-6,- explains the meaning of Christhood, which is an Initiation in Divine Rapture, the God Spell or Illumination. John means God-Endowed (Grace of God) and in the Aramaic text of Jacobites, Nestorians, etc. the word for Baptist is Establisher, Initiator or Lustrator who illumines revealing God within the initiates: the Anointing, Baptizing, etc. is symbolic. To become an Apostle Beloved in Christ, in the True Initiation of Enoch, Elias, and John in the Order of Mt. Carmel, I have experienced the God Spell anointed with the Spirit of Truth, fasted 40 days on Mt. Quilotoa, beside two over 6 months fasts later and realized the Baptism of Living Water, etc. to know what is meant by these Scriptures as to Ascension, Anointing and Baptism of the Holy Spirit.

Again, to illustrate who he was, John quoted another passage in Isaiah: "I am the VOICE OF ONE (God) crying in the wilderness", as the mouth of the Lord shall speak, adding "All flesh is grass...grass withers, flowers fade, but the Word of God stands forever" (Is. 40:3-8), which was illustrated above in Chapter I also, meaning that our flesh dies daily, but Spirit is Eternal.

Thus, John declared he manifested the Word of God, or the Truth, receiving God in him as His Son, first born of the Father, full of Grace and Truth: Jn. 1:11-14. For this he was sent from God (Jn. 1:6), and was named "Grace of God" or the meaning of John in Aramaic, because he, "Grace and Truth (Word of God) came into being by the Anointing Spirit of One who Saves", or "Jesus Christ" translated in meaning from Aramaic, as stated in John 1:17, which is the Key to the Mystery. When the "One" is spoken of as "the Voice of One", "the Saving-Healing One", "the Anointed One", etc. and so often left untranslated, this refers to Oneness in God's Spirit, "I am that I am" or Being ness, which John (10:30) states best saying "I and the Father are One". That Jesus Christ was Spirit, appearing and disappearing among the Disciples of John, he did not leave any question about saying, "Among you stands one whom you do not know."

In Aramaic, as a Peshitta N.T. Lexicon can illustrate, the word for SPIRIT, breath, wind, Vital Principle, Life, heart, Spiritual Being, God, Divine Spirit, Angels and evil spirits or evil powers are all expressed in one word: ROKHA. This will account for a broader scope of interpretation requiring Spiritual Insight. Nature is the system of the earth's laws, everything on earth that is not made by man. As illustrated in the "Our Father" prayer, in Aramaic "Bread" is used to mean food of any kind, as George Lamsa tells in his works, so that Living Bread really means Living Food.

CHAPTER II (1-40)

Your flesh, your bones, your veins and arteries, and the blood flowing in them all came from Mother Earth, from her minerals, greens, vegetables, fruits, and her waters, air, sunshine and all these blessings that we enjoy due to the kindness of Mother Nature. Seeing by our eyes, hearing by our ears, smelling by our nostrils, all are gifts born of colors, sounds and aromas given us by our Mother Earth. The blood that gives us life has its origin in water where ever it is to be found which is the bloodstream of Mother Earth. She fills the oceans, lakes and rivers. Sunshine causes it to evaporate and rise up into the atmosphere as clouds which descend again as the morning dew and beneficial rains that makes vegetation grow, including crops that give us our daily food.

The atmosphere is a blessing that penetrates to the depth of our being, and encloses us like water does a fish, the earth a seed and the air the birds of the sky. Where the atmosphere contains water, it forms the many colored clouds that adorn the heavens with beautiful scenes which may turn into tempests with flashing lightning that often sets fires, and whose deafening thunder may cause a shuddering, shaking, stirring, awakening and reviving of the sleeping earth's topsoil yielding many benefits to growing plants. All of such phenomena in Nature have reason for being because they are necessary and useful, altho as yet, men may not understand or fear them. Where there are changes in temperature within the various layers of atmosphere, violent winds are caused which stir up the stagnant air, filling it with oxygen, even as the fresh breeze scatters the pollen that fecundates the blossoms that make all vegetation fruitful. Likewise, water, which is the basic substance of Nature and the living bloodstream of Mother Earth, flowing within and around her, to be found from the clouds high in the atmosphere which give productive rains and dew to the crystalline well springs of her depths, which gives Life to all that lives on this wonderful planet called earth; the eternal snows that sleep upon and adorn her mountain peaks melt and likewise, drop by drop, gather the precious substance that forms the murmuring streams and brooks that enlarge into imposing rivers that finally flow into lagoons and the rushing sea.

I say it is very true that you are the children of Mother Nature, of the Earthly Mother because from her you received all that you are, all your earthly body just as you received your spiritual body from your Heavenly Father. This fact is as true and undeniable as the truth that a new born babe is the child of his or her mother.

Soil (dust) you are, and Soil you shall become, because from this Earthly Mother you came, and to her each day you shall return, since you are One with the Mother Earth, she is in you and you are in her. Of her you were born, from her you live and to her each day you must return because your body is of her substance and to her substance it returns. Thus, you must honor and keep the wise Teachings that your Mother in Nature yields for you, because no one can attain to perfect health and longevity, nor be happy, but by the faithful observance of the Commandments of your Mother in Nature, loving and serving her with all your strength and all your understanding. To love her and to serve her means to practice and live exemplifying the greatest human virtues based on Love. You are intimately united with Mother Nature because your breath is her breath, your pulse is her pulse and your emotions are her emotions. Your blood is her blood, your flesh is her flesh, your bones her bones and your bowels her bowels. Also, your eyesight, hearing ears and sense of smell are (part of) her eyes, ears and sense of smell.

The Truth of what I am telling you is that whenever your vicious and evil habits harm you, your body or any of the body's organs, by the serious violation of any one of the wise precepts of Mother Nature, you make yourself worthy of painful sanctions in disease, suffering and sorrow. The body you believe to be your own, in reality, is not yours at all, but rather it was loaned to you by Mother Nature, as a tool or instrument of evolution with which your soul will be able to work in the Lord's Laboratory, acquiring experience, knowledge and wisdom. Whenever you suffer from any disease or any pain, this is a sure sign that you have abused your body and disobeyed Mother Nature's Commandments.

In, turn, if at any age you know perfect health, and especially if it be at an advanced age, this is a sure sign that you have kept the Commandments of your Mother in Nature, who thus rewards you with good health and long life. The Truth is that if you abuse your body you are acting in grave violation of Mother Nature's Laws, and in that case you cannot escape punishment, consisting of serious ailments, chronic disease, much suffering and premature death.

Blessed are the children of the Earthly Mother who fully obey her, because she shall caress and cherish them, granting them well being and happiness, material and spiritual prosperity, good health and long life.

If you are suffering chronic illness, disease and pain, I assure you that these evils shall go away as if they vanished by the work of some unknown charm, if you live and work as One with Nature, strictly observing all her Laws, all of which is the reward for returning to the bosom of Mother Nature. Thus, your old age shall be pleasant, without chronic illness, nor pains, enjoying perfect health and long life, filled with happiness and Divine Protection.

The prodigal son who returns to again cling to the bosom of Mother Nature, receiving all her love and protection, shall be protected from attacks of the lawless, accidents, bites of poisonous snakes, ferocious animals, fires, bad harvests, floods, earthquakes and all risks and dangers that plague the rebellious sons who scoff at their own Mother and trample on her commandments. Yet in spite of this rebellion, Mother Nature tenderly loves even these bad children, sacrificing to care for them when they fall ill. This is because only Mother Nature has the Power to Heal us if we get sick. Outside of her, nothing and no one in all the world can heal us, not even the most learned among physicians with all their miracle remedies and formulas, because medicines and remedies never heal, nor can they heal ever. The only thing that CAN HEAL DISEASE or restore health is the STRICT ADHERENCE TO THE LAWS OF NATURE. Due to this cause, acting in violation of her Divine Laws, no scientist will ever discover a miraculous drug (same as poison in Aramaic) that can heal any disease. Blessed are they who are humble and obedient children and obey Mother Nature, because they shall be fondled and protected, safe in her gentle bosom.

Verily I say unto you, Mother Nature never ceases to love her children, altho she is saddened when they are disobedient, becoming ashamed of her laws and abandon her. Great indeed is her Joy when a prodigal son or daughter returns, repents and again receives her embrace. Such is her Love, vaster than gigantic mountains and deeper than the deepest oceans. These penitent children she showers with her blessings, with her gifts and privileges. She cares for and protects them as a hen protects her chickens, as the lioness her cubs. Just as the newborn babe can confide and feels safe in his mother's arms, those who return to the embrace of our loving Mother Nature with absolute faith and trust shall be cared and protected from all evil.

///////////////

Ed. Note: The Living Water of Living Food of Living Trees of the Living Soil is the Natural Healing message of the Eternal Healer, Savior or Jesus Anointed with the God Spell. As revealed already, Life Sciences are Eternal, Paradisian.

CHAPTER III (1-42)

Never shall I tire in repeating that our Mother in Nature tenderly loves her children. Even the most evil ones she loves and eagerly protects in their ignorance after they bring misfortune upon themselves. Nor does she deny her loving protection even to those who insult her, shun her and scorn her. In her loving, gentle and persuasive ways she speaks to them thru the Voice of their Conscience, giving them a feeling of uneasiness in wrong actions so as to convince them that they should return to her gentle embrace in the path of right living. But when her good council fails, as well as her persuasive efforts, the loving and smiling face of Mother Nature becomes solemn, grave and severe. Not accepting her Mercy, they hand themselves over to the Lord of Pain, to the harsh Angel Pain, who thru unbearable but sometimes convincing torment, is sometimes able to make them return to an honorable and decent life, the practice of human virtues achieved thru valiant and honest work.

Angel Pain comes under the symbolic figure of a congenial devil in appearance,- attractive, agreeable, smiling and always happy, of courteous manners, but deep within is mischievous, wicked and criminal. This is why he is known as Beelzebub, who is the Prince of Devils, the most evil of the evil ones. He is a master in setting traps for humans, in weaving fine nets, like a spider's web to catch them like flies. As hook and bait he employs the enticements and weakness of each individual, their most gleeful, merry vices, by which they shall gain painful experience, which contains no motive of vengeance, but is highly educational and instructive in essence coming out of the purest Love. His followers he exposes to grave dangers, serious accidents and calamities without end to make them feel and see the effects of their own vices, and thus, persuade them to abandon them and to return to Right Living.

This Prince of Evil, taking on pleasing raiment and clothed in riches, knows how to tempt and entice each and everyone, using their Desires and whatever their heart is most inclined to. Some followers are best enticed by dazzling Riches, shining gold and silver, splendid palaces with luxurious accommodations; others in turn are most easily tempted by Power, rulership, fame, luxury, titles of nobility, renown and glory, and still others he attracts with lustfulness, sexual orgies, drugs, gambling, riotous living and idle pleasure. Blinded by these alluring wonders, all this splendor, beauty and glory, they soon become caught in the web of Satan.

Once they do become snared these delights are generously provided for their pleasure for a short while, to enjoy to their passionate desire. But then, when they reach the summit of their desires, Satan sends them tumbling down into the deepest abyss of depression. He snatches away all that allured them, - riches, gold, silver, palaces, luxury, fame, sexual pleasure and even their health, giving them a Trip that sends them stumbling headlong down, head over heels, to the uttermost depths of horrible moral depravation, the Trip of Drug Addiction, Drunkenness, sexual orgy, gambling, crime, licentious life of the slothful, and finally ends, landing like social trash and rubbish in slums, hospitals, correctional houses, madhouses, prisons and death in utmost misery.

So many vices have poisoned their organism that their bodies have become a morbid mass of waste matter. Their bodies are full of abominable filth, coming from their riotous and polluting gluttony, intoxicating liquors and narcotic drugs. Their organs are foul with great amounts of accumulated, indigestible and decayed food, converting them into human dung heaps, coming with worms, an infinity of infectious microorganisms, causing even visible plagues of rotting flesh, starting from skin sores, boils, ulcers, tumors and going on to cancer, gangrene and leprosy in the most chronically morbid. It all begins with irregular bowel movements of nauseating stench, telltale filth.

This waste matter thickens, coagulating the blood, giving leukaemia, blood clots or darkens it to form gangrene, varicose veins, and gives forth an appearance uglier and more morbid than the dead, stagnant morass waters of a swamp. The defiled bloodstream scatters its filth and toxins thru-out the organism, infecting it thru-out, the bones, the nerves, veins, beside the flesh, till the most vital organs begin to fail. The bones lose their firmness, becoming fragile, knotty and brittle. (osteoporosis, arthritis, bone cancer) The breathing becomes laborious, at times with gasping asphyxiation. The lungs become perforated and no longer do they function normally. From within the fetid stench comes forth in the breath, vomit, wind and evacuations of the bowels. The eyes lose their brilliance becoming cloudy, glassy, bloodshot or of muddy colors without life and finally become blind partially or completely. Nor do the ears function properly, because their delicate cavities are obstructed with toxic waste, ending eventually with complete deafness. In a similar fashion the keen sense of smell becomes dull and absent.

In a similar way, all the blessings of Mother Nature that the rebellious and incorrigible child originally had, are now taken away: breath, blood, eyes, ears, nose, flesh and sleep. His mind fails, finally becoming mentally deficient or completely insane. Such is the punishment of wicked children who do not heed Mother Nature. Yet, if this obstinate son be sorry for his sins and willingly undo them, returning to his Mother's bosom in Nature, she will greatly rejoice and again receive him with open arms and pardon. All that is needed is that he returns to an honest life of honorable work and right living, without evil habits and vices. Above all, he must keep the Laws of our Creator in the Precepts of Mother Nature, so as to free himself from the clutches of his tormentor, the unappeasable Satan, and his torments, to resist all the temptations with future enticements he may offer. Once the prodigal child proves to Mother Nature that he really is taking life seriously, and makes an effort to regenerate himself, she will afford him every aid within her immense Love for all. As soon as the prodigal son sees himself free from the torments of Satan, he will realize with joy that the only way to free one's self from suffering, is to remain steadfast within the gentle and safe embrace of our loving Mother in Nature, obeying all that she teaches us.

In conclusion, to make it very clear, whenever the erring Son of Adam, or Man, returns to the bosom of Eve, or Mother of all living, forsaking all sin, vices and bad habits of those in Satan's fold, resisting all temptations of the evil one, he shall be emancipated, safe in the embrace of our Mother. For no man can serve two masters. Either he serves God (Spirit, Angels, etc.) and Mother Nature (Ecology, Environment, Paradise), or else you serve Beelzebub and his devils. Behold, I set before you the Way of Life and the Way of Death.

///////////////

Ed. Notes: Adam means red earth, since the Image of the Heavenly Father was formed from the soil, containing earth dust, inflated by the Wind, Breath or Spirit of God to give him Life as a soul. The Heavenly Man (Natura Naturans) gave body, flesh and bone, to the Earthly Man-kind (Natura Naturata) thru Eve, the Mother of all the Living on Earth, our Earthly Mother in Nature. (Genesis 1:27; 2:7,23; 3:19,20, and the multiple meanings of Aramaic words for the above.

CHAPTER IV

All those gathered around John and his Elect Disciples listened to these Words of Wisdom (Gnostic Logos) with wonder, due to his intimate relationship with the Lord. His Teaching or Word was full of Wisdom in Spirit, and with a profound moral significance, spoken with Power and Authority, without hesitancy or unsure statements like those of the Priests and Scribes. So great was the Power of the Lord's Anointed that he inevitably drew a multitude that even with the setting of the sun, they departed not, continuing to sit around him listening and asking him questions.

And they asked him: "Teach us the Laws of Life, explain to us how we may live in harmony with Mother Nature and keep her commandments, because we want to be healed, to be happy and to live long."

The Healing and Saving One answered them: "Verily the Truth is as I tell you: No one can be happy unless they keep the Commandments of Mother Nature."

And the Scribes and Pharisees answered "We do the Commandments in the Laws Moses, our Lawgiver, gave us as they are written in the Holy Scriptures."

And thereupon the Voice of He who Saves and Heals spoke out with vital emphasis and clarity: "Seek not the Law of Life in your Scriptures. Your Scriptures are only a Dead Word in writing, but the Living Law quickens (makes live or enlivens). Surely you know that Moses did not receive his Law in writing, but rather they were of a Living Voice. The Law of Life is the Living Word, of the Living God, to Living Prophets for Living Men, Mankind. The Law is written in the ineffaceable Word in all Living Creation, or Nature, in all that quivers or vibrates with Life from where she speaks forth in thousands of ways. You may learn to hear and read this Law in the Book of Life, the Living Book seen in Nature, the Living Creation: in the herbs when they speak forth with blossoms and aromas; in orchards of fruit trees ripening with delicious fruits, Life speaks to us from the Living Waters in a Voice of Eternal Tenderness. Nature likewise speaks in the crystalline springs that feed streams and rivers, in the oceans that seem to breathe in and out with high and low tides beside their threatening waves. Even the hardest stones are held together due to the vibrant life without which power they would disintegrate like dust. The Truth thus manifest, speaks forth crying out from the stones and solid rocks, (Luke 19:40) as well as the vibrant minerals; from both the animal and vegetable kingdoms; from the seas with multiple named, sized, shaped and colored fishes of the depths, to the heights of heaven from whence come birds to sing among the trees.

Verily, verily I say unto you, Seek the Living Law of Life,

above all, in your very selves, and try to understand and put it in practice; this is the only way to have good health and to be happy. In Truth, all these quivering, vibrating manifestations are closer to God than any "<u>Book</u> of the <u>Dead</u>", whose writings lack Life and are inert. The Living God, in His Infinite Wisdom created the miracle of Living Creation with all that lives, moves and has being, so that by her very Nature she might reveal and teach the Wisdom of her Laws thru thousands of ways and infinite manifestations. (Acts 7:22,38)

In turn, the Creator endowed man with Reason, Intelligence and Wisdom by giving him a share in His Divine Spirit, so that thru enlightened insight he might understand Nature's Living Scriptures and the Living Laws so as to be able to practice them. This is why people should use their intelligence to search out Wisdom in the Laws of Creation because this is the only way they will know what to do to keep them. Woe unto whoever shuts his or her eyes to avoid seeing the Reality of Life, and Woe unto whoever stops up his or her ears to avoid hearing the coming of the unswerving advance of unrestrainable progress. Again, may I reiterate, the Scriptures are the work of erring men, subject to errors of interpretation, while the unwritten Word is a Teaching manifest thru-out all Living Creation, and is God's Work, the only Authentic Scripture found in His Universal Tongue, so as to be without error, Infallible.

Woe unto whosoever prefers to hear the Dead Scriptures of anachronistic papyri and musty manuscripts, to hearing the fresh Living Word that God speaks thru-out the Nature of Living Creation, whispering to all thru infinite ways but with One Tongue within the heart, mind and conscience of each individual. He is not the God of the dead, but of the living.

///////////////// (Read Acts 7:22=Moses)
Ed. Notes: In this 4th Chapter, God's Word spoken thru John reveals that the O.T. Hebrew Scriptures were not given by the Law-Giver or the Living God, but are really taken from the Egyptian "BOOK OF THE DEAD" which contains the Ten Commandments, rituals and all history prior to coming to Egypt back to Paradise. The "Mosheh" is a transliteration from the Greek Moses meaning Law Giver. In John 5:39 we are told to Search these Scriptures, if therein any Life exists... A-Brahm is a Hindu word, "Brahm" meaning God and "A" is First or "Supreme", which by traditions the Jews named "Father of all

who live."

As to "Jesus" in John (Jn. 7:5), even his own brethren did not believe in him! This later was proven by his half-brother when he wrote the Hebrew historical mss. "Protevangelium", (of which the 4 N.T. Gospels are but versions), that this "Jesus" appearing as John Glorified in the Apostles, was the son of Zacharius and Mary born out of wedlock, because Elizabeth was old and barren making Zacharius' priesthood appear fruitless in Jewish tradition. Thus, John was first recorded as the son of Zacharius and Elizabeth, and later claimed to be "Jesus" born of the Holy Spirit to Joseph and Mary. This is why Jews accused "Jesus" of being born in sin, while God spoke thru their Law Giver (Jn. 9:29,34). Every time one prays the "Hail Mary", one acknowledges Mary was big or "Full with Grace" of God, the literal meaning of John, making him as Savior (Jesus) the son of David thru Zacharius an anointed priest (Luke 1:28-32).

When Aramaic was translated into Greek, it began using the word "of", a word non-existent in Aramaic, and this non-existent "of" is given 13 English equivalents. Thus, the Scriptures became even more veiled or mystical. Having spoken a dialect similar to Aramaic (Estonian), I know how deceptive English expressions are compared to Peshitta, or Pure Tongue. If one will retranslate their N.T. Bible stating things without using "of", the Message of the Healing God Spell therein will be discovered. The N.T. written in our hearts tells us that instead of "Tree of Life" it should say living tree, "Water of Life", is living water, "Bread of Life" is living food, "Book of Life" is living book. Deceptive speech gives death to works, since one "lives" by reading "of" them.

When St. John arose from the dead, he had not really been crucified, but the allegory was derived from the fact that in Aramaic "elevate, exalt, lift up and crucify" are one word, Mark 15:25,27; John 19:15; Matt. 26:2, all referring to the Ascension of John "the Baptist" to Savior and Messiah after he lost his head. "When you shall have lifted up the son of man then you shall know that I am he, and that I do nothing of myself but as the Father hath taught me I (in my Apostles) speak: Abide in me and I in you" (Jn. 8:28; 15:4). Even the sea is said to arise or get "High" in a storm (Jn. 6:18) with the same word but in Aramaic one does not mean the sea was crucified. The allegory of John (Apostle) of the N.T. having Salome, his mother, accompany him contemplating the crucifixion comes with John's head being given to Peace unharmed, which is the literal meaning of Salome, relating to Herod's daughter and John's accusations against Herod. John lost his head in holy anger, becoming "mad" raving about Herod's act of incest, but Herod heard him willingly, honoring him as a holy man. (See Mark 6:28; 15:40; 16:1) When the 12 Apostles were sent out they preached God's Kingdom and healed the sick in the Savior's name, and when Herod heard of it he was told THAT JOHN HAD RISEN FROM THE DEAD! (Luke 9:1-8) Thus, the Gnostic First Christians of Mt. Carmel Colleges established an Order in Samaria under St. John. It was a Disciple (Matthew in Aramaic) named Manaen, foster-brother of Herod who went to Antioch (Acts 13:1), Manahen meaning "numbered" or appointed in place of Judas, also called Barnabas, who wrote the First Gospel, and Allegory Key with John's Gospel. He was known as Maen-Andros, founder of the Gnostic Maendeans, Manicheans First Christians of Antioch and Teacher of Basilides who founded a school in Alexandria. In Ephesus he is known as the writer of the Apocalypse, Disciple of St. John (Baptist). Paul gave the single Gospel of Marc John (Marcion) at Pontus who translated it in Greek. Confusion of many untranslated titles gives the illusion that all the mentioned were different people. As Maerinthus it meant Merciful.

This would account for Church Father Irenaeus stating "from 40th to 50th year our Lord taught the Gospel as all our Elders in Asia with John will testify", quoting Polycarp, proving without a doubt the Anointed Savior manifest in John was not executed in 33 A.D. In this Immortal Spirit, and biologically in the flesh and body of John, I continue to teach since I again began writing in English (at Quilotoa, 1945) that the righteous who live not in sin, do not die unjustly early in youth (33 A.D.), but this is the wish of sinners who fear that Karmic Law may be true! Only "He who kills by the sword shall die by the sword",- Law of Karma of Gnostics, from Christianity to Eastern Philosophy.

But after finding life hard hunting fruit of the Locust Tree (Carob in Aramaic) and becoming like Milarepa's "hungry ghosts", John found flesh and blood cannot inherit the Kingdom of Heaven even in Nature. Thus, he began his career as Anointed or Ordained Apostle of God's Word, Logos, giving early Gnostic Christian Vicars or Doctors. Thus, like Buddha's Bhikshus, the Apostles lived on Alms. Yet as told in John 21:23, for near 2000 years (Apoc. 20), I remained patiently to now reveal that mankind does not inherit Fruitful Paradises until he begins to BUILD PARADISES and keep the First Paradisian Law of Life, nourishing from the Living Water of juicy fruits, to get lifted up on High instead of crucified. Serpents of Wisdom shall lift up Paradises in the Desert! (Gnostics, Jn. 3:14)

CHAPTER V -THE HEALING GOD SPELL OF ST. JOHN
Then the Scribes and Pharisees said to him: our forefathers only taught us the knowledge of the Law of the Scriptures. Thus, to read the Law in Natural Phenomena is something new to us since we have neither inherited or learned such a way of interpretation from our elders. Moreover, we ask that you teach us the Law of which you speak, because learning it, we willingly would put it in practice, so we may become healed and be right with God".

The Anointed responded: "Since you only understand the dead Word in the dead Scriptures, your Spirit is dead also, and nothing makes sense, like the blind walking and stumbling in darkness. This is why you cannot even discern a glimmering semblance in the vibrant manifestations of Life in Living Creation.

Verily in truth I tell you that your poring over the Dead Word in musty books and rancid manuscripts has profited you nothing at all, since you have lost sight of the Living Word in the open book of Ever-living Nature in perpetual renovation. The Dead Word, lacking Life, deadens your heart. Since you deny your Heavenly Father in your deeds, no new human virtue can bud or spring forth to make you worthy of Him. Deep in your souls I find only those evil emotions that drag one down to lower passions, great moral sins such as sexual abuse, alcoholism, gluttony, conceit, selfishness and greedy desire for more and more riches, usurping even the little the poor, the aged, widows, orphans and the invalid may have, while their souls cry out to heaven for justice in such abuse. Woe unto those Scribes and Pharisees who do nothing to escape the punishment they deserve. Even your great Commandments tell you, Thou shalt not Fornicate, but you fornicate; Thou shalt not Kill, yet you kill; Thou shalt not bear false witness, yet you falsify; Thou shalt not Hate, but you hate, not only your enemies but even your own brethren. Woe unto you Scribes and Pharisees who do nothing to escape a most certain punishment you deserve.

The Living Truth is that your living bodies were created to be the Sacred Temple of the Living God and your Hearts, His Holy Sanctuary. But when this Temple is defiled and made into the den of dishonest scheming, thieving and abominable practices, the Lord refuses to inhabit therein.

If you want God to dwell within your hearts, along with the angels of His Heavenly Paradise, you must restore immaculate purity in cleanliness within your Temple, which is to say, you must live an honest life, in purity and in morality, without resorting to the evil habits and vices, dedicated to honest and earnest work restoring God's Realm, along with Fasting and Prayer.

///////////////

Editor's Notes on Scriptures continued: Saint John's Gnostic FIRST CHRISTIANS OF ANTIOCH were founded by remnants of a Samaritan ORDER OF MT. CARMEL, also described as the Sons of the Prophets, the Gnostic Essenes, or of the "Good Samaritan" epithet their Savior attached to their pious, dating back to Elias. They were believed to be a "Shoot of the rod of Jesse (father of David, which means Beloved), "on whom the Spirit of Wisdom (Gnosis) shall rest", where the wolf and lamb dwell together, cow and bear feed together and a little child shall lead them, play with a Serpent and put the hand in an asp's hole. They shall not hurt nor destroy life on all God's Holy Mountain, for the earth shall be filled with the Lord's Gnosis...and whom the Gentiles shall seek...They shall trust in God as their Healer, the Lord as their Strength and Salvation. (See Isaiah 11 and 12) The followers of the Savior (Jesus) would be called Jessenes or Essenes as Epiphanius identified them, also saying they wrote the N.T. Gospels and Epistles, just as Church Historian Eusebius also confirms but names them as "Therapeuts" or Healers, which comes from "Jesus" meaning Healer.

The early Church Father, St. Clement of Alexandria, clearly stated, "After the Resurrection the Lord delivered the GNOSIS to James the Just, John and Simon Peter, and they delivered it to the Apostles," proving the so-called Essenes were Gnostics, which the Church later sought to eradicate from their usurped membership. In the "Gnostic Gospel of Thomas", Robert Grant writes, "When such people (Essenes) transferred their hopes from earth to heaven, they created the religious movement known as Gnosticism."

Samaria, properly denominated "Israel", north of Judea, had its temple on Mt. Gerizm which they held holier than Jerusalem of Judea, since they kept to the purest origin of Religion, rejecting the history of bloody wars and conquests made by the Jews, accepting the Five Books of the Lawgiver (Moses) and thus were regarded as heretics by Jews. The Samaritan doctrine accepted the existence of Angels, the Resurrection, that the Messiah would manifest only as a prophet as John Baptist did, rebelled against Jewish dominion and in the temple taught that God's kingdom could not be localized in any earthy State, which coincides with the Essene Gnostics of Mt. Carmel in Samaria. Thus, like Abraham (A-Brahm) they claimed an Eastern origin of their inhabitants, coming from Assyria in 722 B.C. beside thru King David, the Anointed (2 Sam. 23:1) whose son was King over all Israel, and married Pharaoh's daughter, just as Moses was (believed) a son of Pharaoh's daughter, as an Egyptian hierophant, making possible his amassing of wealth and wisdom. "Jesus" tells us, many, but not Jews, are to be saved and God's Kingdom will be given to another nation (Matt. 21:43) and he presented the "Good Samaritan" as his model Healer, showing how his disciples "love one another" (Luke 10:27-37) and also in the case of ten lepers healed, only the Samaritan gave thanks for being healed (Lk. 17:16), illustrating that both Faith and Knowledge are needed to establish God's Kingdom within one.

This should justify our seeking the origin of the Christian Gnostics in Samarian Carmelite Colleges. In our Introduction we have illustrated that Simon Magus, an Essene, became the Disciple of John Baptist, which corresponds to the N.T. "Simon" called Peter, Rock of Faith or Church cornerstone. Simon's arrogance and gaining power over other humans coincides with Simon of Gitta Samaria, both being accused by the Anointed as being of Satan (Mt. 16:23), and named Simon Zealot among the Apostles. Two or more Simons correspond to Simon Magus teaching of reincarnation, the Zealot dying crucified we matched within Josephus' claim, and of Roman Church "Peter", the death being karma from incarnation as Zealot soldier or "living by the sword" as a fisherman of Galilee, and reborn as Simon of Gnosis and Power, educated Greek scholar.

Simon means Sun, and thus as Simon Magus he was known as the "Incarnation of the Great Power" or "Almighty", as to Life on earth, while his consort is Helen which comes from the Greek word for Moon. In Simon's "Great Announcement" mss. (Good News or Gospel) Simon Magus, like "Peter", teaches the fundamental concepts of all the Gospels, especially elaborating his Crucifixion of Simon Zealot, the Galilean, of whom he is the Resurrection (Reincarnation). Likewise to illustrate his Power of Gnosis over all obstacles to Salvation, Simon Magus gives an example from his own life in which he selects as a consort Helen, an abused woman who had to suffer much indignity in this life because she is the reincarnation of Helen of Troy, who Simon rescued from destiny in a brothel. This rescue from abuse and indignity corresponds identically to the Savior of the N.T. who also makes Mary of Bethany his consort in the Love Scene or Anointing as the Savior, heals the woman who has had blood flow (menstruation) for 12 years, and gives John's secret of Living Water (Vitalogy, Dietetic Science of Continence) to the Samaritan woman with 5 husbands, who becomes the earliest evangelist teaching about the Savior (John 4:9-42), just as Gnostics claimed. This is the Gnostic Mar-iame who gives the Gospel account of the Crucifixion (dramatized by Simon Magus) to James, and other Apostles not present, accounting for Gnostic works abounding with early teaching of Women's Liberation illustrated in dialogues of 3 or more Marys, Sophia, Martha, Salome, etc. giving physical, mental and spiritual concepts of "Mother of God" or Love, "the most Spiritual among Disciples" or "Lady Elect" of John. While the Sun is the King of Heaven, in Simon's Aeonology, the Moon is the "Queen of Heaven" and the 12 signs of the Zodiac will be represented by 12 Apostles who rule aspects each of us are born under in the 12 months of the year.

 Not only is the dialogue going on in Martha-Mary, Virgin Mary-Mary Magdalene, Sophia-Helen questions, but we also have the multiple Simons controversy engendered by gossip, taking of sides by interested parties and resultant myth. Simon, the Wonder-Worker of Samaria (Israel) is mistaken by Zealot-Galileans to be the very Simon that was their leader, and thus, like the resurrected Alexander Josephus tells about the exploits in his History, this rapidly develops into the Resurrected Simon Zealot, Risen King of Israel. Already, he has become famous for being "Almighty" in Power of Miracles, which Simon recorded in what is known as "The Lost Gospel According to Peter," the original from which other Gospel versions were built around. In named Apollos, a disciple of John the Baptist, according to Jean Steinman's it Simon cries out: "My Power, my Power, thou hast forsaken me", and immediately he is taken up after crucifixion, Petronius with guards keep watch over the rock sealing the tomb but a great light came and the crucified "reached unto heaven and beyond", so Petronius and Pilate agree to tell no one of the escape. The pseudo-Alexander likewise acquired fame by telling of how he escaped from supposed Alexander's tomb, but Simon sought no lie, because in truth he was a reincarnation of the Galilean hero, just as Helen had been Mary, Simon's wife, and before that Helen of Troy. But after the Fall of Jerusalem, the Savior of Israel and Jews, was no longer a valid Passport for Welcome,- so why not be born again in a new mission, avoiding much of the accusation and being found out, like "Alexander"?

Paul is generally agreed to have written before the 4 Gospels were known, being the earliest source of the Vision of Christ experience. Paul like Simon of Samaria know nothing about the Savior's life except being born of the Holy Spirit. Paul says that after his Gnosis experience, when Christ began to dwell in him, for 3 years he did not talk to any of the Apostles, "I conferred not with flesh and blood, neither went I to Jerusalem to them that were Apostles before me, but went away to Arabia (Gal. 1:16) contradicting the writer of Acts (9). Now, this gives a clue, since Dositheus was from Arabia, his disciples lived like the Essenes and both Simon and Dositheus were Disciples of John Baptist. The "Wise Men" were supposed to have come from Arabia according to Justin Martyr, and this has been believed to be a source of Essene Gnosticism. But when Paul seeks to commune with priests in Jerusalem, he takes on the reputation as a heretic due to his doctrine against Jewish rituals.

Baur and his followers in the Tubingen school have demonstrated the theory that Simon Magus is simply the legendary symbol for Paul, giving clues to the multiple Simon drama. Peter and Paul are said to have quarrelled in Antioch, never to meet again (Gal. 2:9-14), dramatizing his own internal conflict or schizophrenia. No longer is he merely the follower of John Baptist and Ebionite Jews, but as he discovers his name Simon to mean Sun, among the Greeks he might be considered Apollo,- Apaulo, or Paul. He now shaves his head and beginning with Priscilla and Aquila he acquires his new name from Apollo (Acts 18:18-26). Paul's Epistle to the Hebrews according to

Menequez "is a converted disciple of Philo of Alexandria" and is named Apollos, a disciple of John the Baptist, according to Jean Steinman's book "St. John the Baptist". All this correlates in identity to Simon, the Sun, Samarian Wonder-Worker, who also studied in Alexandria, taught at Antioch, gave his Gospel to Marcion at Pontus, and thus after Ephesus, eventually arrives in Rome. This reconstructs how Simon, in Luke's Acts is transformed into Paul, which in Rome is identified as both Simon Peter and Paul, altho contained in one person, and giving the Peter and Paul founding of the Roman Church with Simon's origin as heretic erased appearing as Peter, meaning Cornerstone of the Christian Church. The Gnostics not only had their Mysteries taught by Allegories, but the New Roman Church, out for political imperial gains, also interpolated Scriptures to hide their Gnostic origins.

Of great importance is this fact that the whole structure of the Church is supposed to rest upon Apostolic succession, with Simon Peter as the cornerstone, thru whom the approved N.T. Canon in Scriptures, doctrines, and authority has been transmitted, and supposedly the Gnostic Christians lacked this causing their deficiency. However, the Gnostics had proof and traditions just as authentic if not more so. Another of the Samaritan Gnostics who also taught at Antioch, and who's doctrine resembled Simon Magus so that Mead considered him Simon's teacher, was Menander, Maenandros (Man, Mani, Manas, Manda all meaning Gnosis and Andros meaning man, son, so combined becomes God-Man or son of Truth-Spirit). He thus gave origin to later Manicheans, Mandeans and the Gnostic First Christians of St. John. John the Baptist was a strange anomaly in being a son of a priest who rejected the exercise of his priesthood in the Temple, which shrouded John's youth in mystery. Zacharias was not of the House of David, being of Aaron lineage, so that out of Zachary's desire to have his son rule Israel, he put John's legal custody under Joseph of Galilee, who he marries to the 14 year old Mary, Mother of Zachary's child (as told in the Protevangelium), because his wife is barren. Thus, thru Joseph, the Savior is the son of David and thru Zachary a priest, and the life of fasting and fruit diet yielded the Chief Prophet, Anointed in the Spirit of God. When Maenandros was teaching in Asia, Ephesus, he was known as Cerinthus (Merinthius by others) and after a long Gnostic career he saw how the Roman Church greedily usurped power, and so prophesied in the Apocalypse, "And in her (Rome symbolized as a Babylon harlot) was found the blood of prophets and of saints and all who were slain on earth. The Roman Church has robbed the earth of the true saints, prostituting Truth in Spirit, by standing alongside the "Merchants of earth", first accepting their living spirit to gain membership, but crucifying, burning and martyring them (like Joan of Arc burnt as a heretic and then made saint), if not denying they were Christians even (as with early Gnostics). So it was with John Apostle, who Gnostics insisted wrote the Apocalypse, beside developing the "Gnosis" in John's Gospel and Epistles. "The John Book", an early Mandean Scripture states: "After the death of John (Baptist), the world will fall a prey to error. The Roman Christ shall overthrow the peoples, the 12 seducers shall travel the world thru-out...corrupt John's sayings, pervert the Baptism of the Jordan, distort the words of truth and preach fraud and malice thru-out the world". This states clearly what the Apocalypse says about Rome, and was accepted (interpolated)! The Gnostics KNEW what Scriptures they had written, and clearly illustrated the original versions of their writings, while the Roman Church relied on Faith in a mythical tradition of Popes, claimed infallible, as the word of God. The Gnostics did not need to defend doctrine by violence, being popular for their Wisdom. Rome had no recourse but accept their Scriptures, interpolated to Roman interpretation, and ruthlessly destroying all signs of their source.

The writer of the N.T. Gospel of Matthew can be traced to Basilides, Gnostic Christian Doctor of Alexandria. Basilides is historically the first writer of Christian Scriptural exegesis, having written 24 books of Commentaries on Hebrew Scriptures, and thus the only person in his time thus capable of taking all the Old Testament prophecies about the Messiah, and integrating them in his version of the Gospel history of Christ. Otherwise, we might have had a Greek or Aryan Wise Men's version of a Savior. He said his doctrine was first revealed by Jesus to Matthias after the Resurrection, yet his teacher was the Gnostic Maenandros, and having studied at Antioch with Simon, Marcion the writer of the original Gospel of Mark, and other great Gnostic Doctors, developed the elaborate Alexandrian theory of Gnosis.

Valentinus is known to have written a Gospel, and for some

reason he was the Greatest of Gnostics of impeccable moral character. To the end he persevered in conciliatory efforts to gain tolerance for the Gnostic viewpoints, but Rome refused to give him recognition as Bishop of Alexandria, in spite of spending years in Rome making a complete elaboration of all previous scriptures and history of the Church acceptable to Rome known as the Acts of Apostles and the Gospel of Luke. Unexcelled in knowledge of other Gnostic sects and the Gnosis of each, yet willing to compromise for a share in recognition by Rome, his pearls were cast only to be trampled on after usurpation by interpolations stating that First Christian Gnostics differed from the mentioned Christian Apostles.

Oddly enough, of all the "Acts of the Apostles" documents in existence, only the part having to do with Simon Peter and Paul was considered canonical, showing how the Roman Church favored only its own tradition of Peter leading the Apostles in everything as their Prince and Bishop, hardly giving mention to the Bishop of Jerusalem, James the Just. Perhaps this may be due to seeking equality with the Gnostic John which in the N.T. might be interpreted that the Beloved Disciple would succeed all the Apostles, giving Simon part as a pupil and pastor of Christ's fold, and "John should never die, but so I will have him remain till I come" (Jn. 21:16-23), just as the Apocalypse obviously condemns Rome as a Babylon harlot, honoring only the 7 Churches of Asia. G.R.S. Mead tells us that the earliest collection of Gnostic Acts of Apostles is that of a certain Leucius, surnamed Charinus, a disciple of John. James held that Leucius (Leukios) who wrote various Gnostic Acts, including those giving the activities and viewpoints of John, Andrew, Thomas beside Peter and Paul. Robert Grant thought Theudas was a name interpreted as Luke, as we do. Valentinus is claimed to have his witness in the tradition of the Gnosis in "Thadeus" as Matt. 10:3 spells it, "Theodas" by others or Theo-Deus (Greek-Roman) meaning God's God just as Elijah (Elohim-Jehova) was said to be God's God for John the Baptist. Basilides had said a "Matthias" (Aramaic for Disciple) had received his Gnosis from Jesus after the Resurrection, and he was a student of Glaucias (G. Laucias) and associate of Peter, tho Basilides was a disciple of Saturnius and Maenander, earliest Doctors at Antioch, and he was the teacher of Valentinus.

Marcion, the author of the N.T. Gospel of Mark (Marc-John),

son of the Bishop of Pontus, and a Man of Letters according to Jerome and Augustine, while Epiphanius wrote "Marcion's followers were to be found thru-out the whole world in his time" when the Church of Rome was unknown. Yet Tertullian thought he was "the most dangerous heretic of his day", and taunted Marcion for not putting his name on his Gospel, but he answered that it was not his to put his name on it, for he had only translated into Greek the Aramaic Gospel Paul used at Pontus. Mark's Gospel is about the Crucifixion, and with it the Epistles of Paul, which illustrates Simon Peter's Gnosis, identify Simon (Sun) with Paul (A-Paulo). This is identical with Marcion's doctrine that Father, Son and Holy Spirit are not people, Holy Spirit being Mother of God, in Christ of an incorruptible and immutable body of Light of Ethereal Fire. Jesus means Healer and son of David means son of the Beloved, knowing nothing of Jewish genealogies.

When Papias claimed Mattheu (Matthias) composed the Oracles (Gospels) in 149, if we would fully translate it, it only meant the Disciples composed the Oracles. These Gnostic Christians of St. John are known as Mandeans in Iraq and Iran, but in Syria-Palestine they were called Nassarenes, Nass-Aryans, meaning non-Judaic inhabitants (just as Samarians and Galileans were from Assyria) who followed the Wisdom-Serpent sect, whose Savior said "Be wise as Serpents". They follow the Gospel of Peter and honor the Anointed wrote Theodoret. Before being called Christians the N.T. Bible called them Nassarenes: Act. 3:6, 4:10, 6:14, 22:8, 24:5, 26:9, Jn. 18:5, Luke 18:37, Mt. 2:23, 10:47, 26:71. At the time of Christ there was no town of Nazareth, unknown to Josephus, but established by myth.

CHAPTER VI (1-20)

Overcome the temptations of Satan! Conquer the evil passions! Make war unceasingly against all vices and uproot them from your lower emotional make-up by concentrating on the opposite virtues to replace sins that once tormented your soul. If you are an alcoholic, your Salvation is to be found in total abstinence and dwelling in sobriety. If one is a sexual offender, one's mind must be filled with the benefits of purity and continence. To obtain power and protection in your self conquest you must seek out the Lord and pray for Faith. Purge your moral structure thru abstinence from vices and evil habits, starting with the most gross, such as sexual abuse and alcoholism. Rigorous fasts and devoted prayer will greatly help one put up an overwhelming fight against Satan. The Truth of the whole matter is that Satan and all his evils can only be cast out from the depths of your being thru FASTING and PRAYER, which like the warm sun that drives away the cold, can remove all these evils.

Flee to the solitudes of the unspoiled country where it is the easiest to fast and pray, meditating in contact with Nature. There amongst the living green surroundings contemplate the magnificence of Nature, the earth and the heavens, and God's great Wisdom in creating all these wonders. Above all meditate upon the greatness of human virtues in good that I shall be revealing to you.

Remember that watching over you in secret is God who greatly rejoices when He sees in your heart the sincere desire and your effort to be good and practice human virtue. He will encourage you onward with the blessings of good health, abundance, honor and eternal happiness. But you must have Faith in the most powerful weapon that exists for the casting away of Satan, which is devoted prayer and dedicated fasting. With these two weapons you can free yourself from the evil one and make clean your being, physically and spiritually, making your Temple a worthy Sanctuary of the Lord, so that his Angels may serve you. Truly, truly I tell you, without Fasting and Prayer you shall never be free from Satan, who manifests in your evil habits and vices, in your disease, pains and mental depression. Only Fasting and Prayer can make clean your Temple, enabling you to live an honest, honorable, pure and holy life dedicated to making better the lives of all and especially your own thru WORK. The Heavenly Father shall be pleased to witness such efforts and shall shower all his kindness and blessings upon you and fill you with joy and happiness.

Yet, this I require of you, that you FAST and PRAY devotedly, for this is your Way of Emancipation from all your conflicts and afflictions materially, morally, emotionally and so many other ways they make torment of human life. Then shall the Spirit of God descend upon you and dwell in your heart. You shall be illumined, anointed with Heavenly Enlightenment, and God's Angels shall aid you in finding the fundamental elements in Nature that can heal your body and soul. (Mt. 17:19, Lk. 4:2, "Do penance", not just repent: Mt. 3:2, 4:17)

Seek the fresh pure air of the forests, fields, mountains or the seashore. Verily I tell you, air is the most essential food for man. You can go many days without eating, but a few moments without air will leave you life-less. Take off your shoes and clothing so that the pure air can bathe all your skin. This air bath should be taken as often as possible because since the beginning of time the skin has had the environmental requirement of being bathed with pure air. Practice deep breathing, embracing the Angel of Air within your lungs allowing deep penetration so that it will charge your blood with Life Energy (Prana) and distribute the healing qualities. In this way, the Pure Air Angel can cleanse your blood and every cell of your body, eliminating all the accumulated wastes and toxins which are the very cause of the diseases and aches that trouble you. Just as air and fire are both necessary to burn bad smelling refuse, so air and heat are necessary for the internal combustion of the fetid wastes even in your body so that bad breath can be made fragrant again. Verily, verily I tell you, no man can find himself in God's Presence unless the Wind of God's Wisdom allows him to do so. God Presence is only achieved thru a thorough Physical and Moral Purification. No man can enter the Paradise Realm of God unless he is born again of this Baptism of the Wind Angel of Breath, the Spirit in Truth, to cleanse his body and soul.

///////////////

Ed. Notes: Words were concealed in meaning in translations of the Bible. All of the HEALING GOD SPELL was contained in the Aramaic originals of the Bible Christians now use, but because Truth in the Spirit of God did not dwell in the vehicles of translation, they could not fully grasp and convey the depth of God's Word. Only realizing that "Rokha" in Aramaic can be used to mean Air, the Vibration of Love, Heart, evil spirit or power, temper, pride and rheumatism, one soon realizes how to contemplate for the Spirit in Words, the symbolic or allegorical Truth, rather than man's limited understanding of copied words.

CHAPTER VII (1-28)

After the embrace of the Angel of air, wind and breath, seek the embrace of the Angel of Pure Waters. Take off your footwear and other clothing (if you have clothed again) and again in the nude totally submerge your body in this liquid substance, that you may be Baptized with the Holy Spirit of Water, cleansing and activating your skin and internal organs. The Truth is obvious that the Pure Water Spirit can purify every cell of your body, to cleanse it of the wastes and toxins eliminated from its depths thru the skin pores. Just as the rapid waters of a stream or river may be used to wash clean our clothing, the lively moving current and our living movement in the waters (swimming or splashing) shall cleanse and purify your bodies of much of its waste matter.

So great is the Spirit of Water Power, when not left stagnant to become stale and unhealthy in swamps, ponds and dead seas, that in the free rapid flow of streams and rivers, where it may be oxygenated, purified and made healthy as it continually beats upon the rocks and churns around here and there, not only providing man with his bodily need for water, but gives him the power to move huge mills that grind wheat for the daily bread of worldlings.

However, it is not enough to clean the vessel of life only on the outside. Of even greater importance is it that the Power of Water cleanse within. (Matt. 23:25, Luke 11:39). Truly I tell you, just as the Angel of Water cleanses and quickens life on the surface of the body, in the same way Pure Living Water quickens, vivifies and purifies the innermost cells of the body. You should partake of LIVING WATER in preference to any drink since the Spirit or Angel of God quickens or gives the Life Principle to this water, making it unsurpassed by other liquids artificially prepared by man.

Partaking of this River of Living Water, you shall not thirst because this is the Living Tree yielding Living Fruits that are LIVING FOOD indeed, both Healing and Life Giving. (Apoc. 22:1,2,14,17; Jn. 4:13, 6:33-64; Gen. 1:29, 3:22) Only by always partaking of this Living Water shall your digestive organs and innermost cells be cleansed and remain pure, eliminating intestinal fever, indigestion and constipation in the intestines. This is why I have formulated such parables to explain that it is necessary to make clean the inside of your vessel first with the Baptism of Water made Living by the Holy Spirit of God, which is much more important than merely washing the surface of the body, for the source of wastes eliminated by the skin is inside. Thus, I have said also that those who clean the outside leaving the inside filthy are like the whited sepulchres which appear clean and holy on the outside, but within are filled with the abominable corruption of the dead. Truly, truly I repeat, that of utmost importance is it that you be Baptized with Pure Living Water to receive the embrace of the Angel of the Holy Spirit, within and outside, the water within and outside your body, thru and thru, freeing you from the deposits and accumulations of infectious waste matter that gives cause for disease.

However, when it is necessary to remove intestinal wastes by washing, make or obtain an enema catheter and water receptacle, and place the water receptacle high enough so the water flows down thru the tube and catheter in thru the anus with enough force to penetrate far enough to loosen up the intestinal wastes. The water should be purified and warmed by the sunlight. One may add a bit of honey or the essence of healing herbs to disinfect and neutralize the evil smelling impurities. To facilitate the penetration of the catheter into (or up thru the loop of the anus, if it is a long and flexible one) one can apply olive oil to it. Let the water remain within as long as possible so as to soften, loosen and remove the wastes adhering to the intestinal canal, mentally directing the Angel of Pure Water to clean well the bowels, freeing them of the impurities that poison the bloodstream and the most vital organs causing their dysfunction giving rise to disease, pain and premature death. Then let the dirty water escape removing all the fetid smelling filth. You will be amazed to see with your own eyes and smell with your own nostrils the fetid abominations that so long have remained stored in your bowels.

The days that you fast use this internal intestinal bath repeatedly, and one should make holy one day each week as the Lord's Day (Sunday) with a complete rest, fasting, since this is the secret to a long life, to good health even at an advanced age, and everlasting happiness. However, the enema need only be repeated until the wash water no longer removes decayed, rotten or hard deposits of a fetid smell. Each time you participate of the external and internal bath, receiving the full embrace of the Angel of Pure Water, make it holy giving thanks to the Lord, God, for He has thus shown mercy on you and freed you, forgiving many sins which you committed against Mother Nature.

Unless you become fully baptized, pure and worthy in body and soul, the Angel of the Holy Spirit in Living Water shall not grant you passage thru the path within the gates of Paradise to live in Highest God Presence. If you have the will power to persevere in your New Covenant with the Lord, in not committing sin against Mother Nature, the Holy Spirit in Wind and Water shall serve you thru-out all your life, that you may live peacefully, enjoying good health, success, longevity and an Everlasting Joy in Living.

////////////////

Ed. Notes: The N.T. Bible's Gospel of John contains all of this in essence in that in Samaria the Savior establishes Living Water as the Fountain of Life Everlasting, then revealing that it did not only satisfy thirst but also it was Living Food cast down from Heaven, which he named as Paradise in his exaltation (crucifixion), as well as show how living water came from the fruits of Paradise when used for living food (or "bread") and that this was the very essence his body and blood consisted of in the Lord's Supper. John's first Epistle 3:9, as well as Matt. 19:12, reveal that the Savior's Message on Life also is the Dietetic Science of Continence, eliminating seminal and menstrual losses, like eunuchs the seed abideth within, which distinguishes the human Gods from Satan's offspring. The author of John's Gospel in the 1st Century was Maenandros who said his interpretation of the Baptism gave internal purification enabling Enlightenment so that one rises from the dead in this very life, "to never grow old or thus become immortal", and thus each of us can become a Savior, a Christ anointed with God's Spirit and a conscious Logos. In fact, Gnostic Christians, unlike the 4th Century Organized Church of the Roman Empire, held strict abstinence from wine, flesh foods and marriage, preferring uncooked nourishment, as the Gnosis or Truth of their Doctrine.

Now, the original "Doctrine of the Twelve Apostles" or "Didache" which dates back to the "First Christians of Antioch", contemporary to N.T. Bible originals, agrees with our God Spell revelation. It begins,- "Behold, I set before you the WAY OF LIFE and the WAY OF DEATH", quoting Jeremiah 21:8, followed by the statement that the Way of Life is first to Love God and second to love one another as one loves oneself: that which you would not have done unto you, do not to another. Jeremiah contains much of our Healing God Spell: 10:10, The Lord is the true God for he is a Living God and Everlasting King; 17:7-14, The Blessed "shall be like a tree planted by the waters, spreading roots out by a stream and is not afraid of heat, it's leaves remain green ever never fearing a year of drought and never ceasing to fruit...Those who leave the Lord, leave this Fountain of Living Water. This Living Lord shall heal me, this Living God shall save me, from Him alone I receive Praise; 7:5-22, "You are the Temple of the Lord, if you amend your Ways...Lying words cannot profit...Has this Dwelling called by My name become a Den of thieves...Neither did I command you holocausts and bloody sacrifices when I brought you out of Egypt."

"The Doctrine of the 12 Apostles" states in its Seventh Commandment: "You shall baptize in the Name of the Father, the Son and the Holy Spirit with Living Water...Before partaking of Baptism, all participants, the baptizer and baptized, must first fast in preparation." Afterward the partaking of food and drink in the Agape is described with the Thanksgiving, which one can be sure ritualistic organized churches will only translate to fit their tradition. However, Dead Bread and Alcoholic Spirits can only give forth Insanity and Death, the attributes of their prepared ingredients. Wine does not keep long unless preserved by fermentation giving alcohol (also used to preserve tissues that would rot otherwise) and such "spirits" bring on possession by evil spirits or insanity. Bread is disintegrated grain requiring removal of essential living enzymes and vitamins to keep long and killing heat to bake. The fact that bread means food in Our Lord's Prayer, and if wine were made anew or fresh in Christ's return to be with us in His Paradisian Kingdom, with Life enzymes and vitamins, should alert us to the fact that our Lord's Supper is to be seen in a bunch of grapes for breaking bread and clenching the grapes over the chalice gives instant wine without fermentation. Moreover, the Roman Church knew that if they revealed the true Holy Eucharist, it would reveal that John Baptist, Beloved Son of God, was the Savior, since he NEVER ATE BREAD nor Partook of Wine, and the foretold Unbloody Sacrifice would be the Holy Communion with Living Saints and would be like taught by the original Gnostic Christians of Saint John. Instead the Roman "Savior" is celebrated with Dead Bread and Alcoholic Spirits to commune with dead Saints and a crucified Savior, who died so we might be forgiven in our way of sin. A god that died is a dead god!

Meditate on the Law of the Lord day and night, be like a tree planted on a stream that brings forth fruit in due season, whose leaves fall not off and whatsoever you begin you accomplish: For the Lord watches over the Way of the Righteous, but the Way of the Unrighteous shall perish. (Psalms 1:1-6, 82:6, Mt.7:14, Jn.1:7)

CHAPTER VIII (1-9)

To complete the Joy of Living close to Mother Nature, she holds for you yet another Angel: the Angel of Sunlight. For the Angels of Air, and of Water and of Sunlight are brethren, and always work together to accomplish the most. Holy likewise, is the embrace of all of them, to be seen in the many blessings we derive from them as Mother Nature and the Heavenly Father intended to provide. So along with the embrace of the Angels of Air and of Water, receive the embrace of the Angel of Sunshine, prudently for short intervals at first and increasing the time until you are fully accustomed. As you enjoy the warm sunshine breathe deeply, filling your lungs with sun-ladened air and charging your blood with Solar Energy which not only heals, but purifies the body of evil smelling wastes. Just as darkness flees with the appearance of the sun, so also shall the darkening murky corruption giving forth evil stench and gloom within disappear when Solar Power enters within our organism, causing each cell of the body to vibrate and radiate with an illumined aura reflecting one's health potential and vitality. On the days that you fast you will find it most beneficent to also receive the Baptism of Fire for purification, because then one best receives its power, not being burdened with digestion. Otherwise the Sun Angel's embrace is best utilized an hour before eating, or two hours after the mid-day meal. Verily, verily I say unto you, unless you are fully Baptized and born again, or continually renewed, of the Holy Spirit in Heavenly Fire, one is not ready to receive God's Presence within to make earth Paradise.

CHAPTER IX (1-19)

When your body is defended by the 3 flaming swords of these 3 Angel Brethren, Air, Water and Sunlight, it becomes fortified against any sort of invasion, so that Satan shall be aghast and flee as fast as he can go. This is because when your Temple is pure, orderly, sunlit and sweet scented thru the godly living conduct of the soul dwelling therein, it means the end to Beelzebub, just as days of hot sunshine bring an end to snow. When the Angel Brethren, Air, Water and Sunshine are in possession of your body, they give it a thorough internal

The Healing God Spell of Saint John

cleaning to even the least accessible recesses, putting its entire in perfect order, because henceforth the true masters and lords shall be in authority and re-establish rule in their castle. Just as thieves flee from an abandoned house with the coming of the true owner in authority, one by the door, another by a window, and the third by road, each from where he is found and whither he is able, even so shall all devils,- which are none other than filthy habits, immoral conduct and sins against Mother Nature,- flee from the Temple of the Lord with the return of the 3 Angel Brethren. That they shall flee by doors and windows is to say that the toxic waste substances will be eliminated from your body thru the pores of the skin, mouth, nose, bowels, urinary channels and every means possible. Like a brisk and efficient broom sweeps clean, so shall all the filth and rubbish be swept out from your organism removing the infecting and contaminating materials with their toxins and stench, and once this house-cleaning is complete, it shall again be clean and breathe forth the fragrance of purity like the blossoms of fruit orchards.

When all your sins and uncleanliness are gone, your blood shall become pure as the bloodstream of Mother Nature, known to us in the pure crystalline water of streams, foaming and racing down from the mountains to quench the thirst of fertile river valleys that yield human sustenance. Also you shall witness the worst corruption in abominable filth come out from within your bowels, skin eruptions, boils, and in many ways visible to your eyes, smelled by your nose and removed by your hands. But after the necessary purging of wastes from all your cells, you are surely going to have vibrant health and be full of vital energy. Your flesh shall become pure as the flesh of the ripening fruit among green leaves of the trees and your body and breath shall breathe forth an aroma, fragrant like the blossoms in Paradise.

Then shall your tired eyes with which you behold your surroundings become rested and be restored to their former greater power of vision. Thru an intricate network of nerves, your eyes are in constant contact with, beside reflecting the state of, every part of your body, so that if your body is clean and healthy, your eyes shall be clear and bright like the sun shining in a blue sky, and act like a wise healer capable of announcing full recovery of health. But if the reverse is true, or your body is toxic, functioning badly and illness lies ahead for you, your eyes shall become dim, dull and dirty, of poor vision or even have cataracts and finally turn blind. These impurities are known to accumulate to make even the lens unclear, the iris color spotted and muddy and the whites loose their sparkle. Verily I tell you, if Light is in your eyes, then in Oneness the body is wholesome, but if the eyes show wickedness, the body is full of disease. (Luke 6:42, 11:34: The eye is one, with body). Applying some local remedy, or medicine to the eyes can never heal them, or the dysfunctions in other parts of the body they represent, since disregarding the oneness of the whole, only worsens the part treated. Only the Integral practice of Natural Hygiene can restore perfect vision. Likewise with the healing of the physical body the soul (psyche) shall become pure and lightsome, because the body and soul are also intimately joined, all in one whole. Only then shall the Angel of the Holy Spirit in Mother Nature clothe you with a clean white garment among those worthy to be received into the Higher Heavenly Hierarchy.

CHAPTER X (1-26)

Verily, verily I tell you, only with the loving Grace of Mother Nature, or true Natural Living, can anyone realize the Supreme Attainment, which is to become one with God, by becoming one with All. Remember the experiences of childhood to better understand what I say. When a little babe your mother nursed, bathed, clothed, rocked your cradle and taught you to walk your first steps. When you had grown, your father took charge of you teaching you his work. He took you with him to his work, to the fields or to his workshop, and taught you to work beside him, just as his father had taught him before he became a skilled and capable master of his work. When your father saw that his son understood his teaching and did his work well, he gave him all he possessed that his beloved son may use this to continue the work of the father.

The same is true with the Sons of the Heavenly Father. Mother Nature rears and takes care of them while they grow strong, teaching, instructing and disciplining them for their good and evil actions. Then when they are ready, she sends them to work with the Heavenly Father. The Divine Father's garden and workshop covers the whole surface of our planet earth. This in fact is a vast University of the Heavenly Father, in which He educates his student body on earth. When they, in turn, possess the needed preparation and maturity, He turns over the Direction of the Universe to continue the Work of the Father thru-out the Heavens, thus realizing the intimate Oneness of the Heavenly Father with Son. This is the Way of Human Unfoldment, the budding, blossoming and fruiting of the Divine Life which is never cut short or interrupted (as often it seems) but endures forever in glorious and triumphant Eternity.

Blessed is the youthful adolescent who willingly obeys his Mother, following her advise and teachings, for soon, at his early age, he shall be able to join in his Father's Divine Labor. Blessed is the youthful adolescent who willingly obeys his Father complying with his wise instruction, so as to become a Good Worker, a Model Citizen, righteous, honest, hard working, generous, kind and noble. This, then is what is meant by the Commandment: "Honor Thy Father and Thy Mother, which is rewarded with Abundance, Happiness and Longevity. Remember well this commandment all your life, ever honoring and keeping the wise Laws of Mother Nature, for this is the only way to lasting Happiness, Higher Attainment and Heavenly Blessings here, now and forever.

By ever loving and honoring your Mother in Nature, you are also loving and honoring your Cosmic or Heavenly Father, Who, well pleased, shall love and honor you with His Blessings. Now, the Heavenly Father is Supreme and Almighty, infinitely greater than all our worlds and their inhabitants, just as Mother Nature is the Mother of all that live including all mothers. Truly, truly I tell you, so great is their love that there is no one, no father and no mother capable of loving us as much as our Heavenly Father and Mother in Nature. Infinitely greater is the Wisdom in the Word of the Heavenly Father, and the Commandments of Mother Nature, than all the teachings and laws that our worldly fathers and mothers have given us. It follows that infinitely greater is the worth of the inheritance with which our Heavenly Father and Mother in Nature shall reward to those who keep their Commandments, than any possible inheritance our worldly parents can leave for us.

Likewise, thou shalt love one another, as true brethren, because your true brethren are those who keep the Commandments, doing the Will of our Heavenly Father and Mother in Nature, rather than those who mock and scoff at their Laws, even if they be our brethren in flesh. I tell you truly, your

True Spiritual Brethren (and Sisters) shall always keep the Laws of the Heavenly Father and Mother Nature, living ever in the Divine Will. And these Spiritual Brethren and Sisters shall love you infinitely more than your brothers and sisters in flesh who rebel against keeping the Lord's Commandments. For since the days of Cain and Abel, when brothers by blood transgressed against God's Will, breaking His Law, the Brotherhood of Man was destroyed. Brothers do unto brothers worse than they do unto strangers often. Therefore, Love your True Spiritual Brethren and Sisters who live in God's Will infinitely more than carnal brothers and sisters who do not. (Lk. 8:2, 14:26; Mk. 10:29; Mt. 19:5)

CHAPTER XI (1-31) THE HEALING GOD SPELL OF ST. JOHN
Verily, verily I say unto you, the law of Love is the Greatest and most important of all the Universe. All that is or exists is subject to Love's Law. Love is God, the Father of All; Love is Nature, the Mother of All, and thus, their Children are Love.

The whole Universe, the earth, moons, suns, stars, planets of the Heavens are inseparable in the Oneness: only thru such Oneness can Cosmos Live and have Being, just as your heart, stomach, liver, lungs, blood and bones of your body are inseparable in their Oneness to be able to exist and live, since Love is the Law that holds everything together in Oneness. The Heavenly Father, the Archangels, the Angels, All of the Heavenly Hierarchy and all of Humanity existing on earth, as well as beings on other planets are ONE, held together by a powerful attraction and cohesion, magnetized by the lodestone of Love. For the Heavenly Father lives in his Sons and Daughters, and these Sons and Daughters live in their Parents. One cannot have Being without the other. The Father exists because Sons and Daughters exist, and They have Being because the Father has Being.

God being Love, humans are also Love, because the Spirit in humans is a portion of God. That the Spirit in mankind might act on the physical plane, or in matter, Spirit had to manifest, materializing on that plane of action. So to function on this earthy plane, the Spirit had to clothe itself with earth elements which as a whole compose Mother Earth. Since Love is the Supreme Law of our Being, keep it with all the Power and Understanding given you. Love the Heavenly Father as He Loves you, and Love one another as you love yourselves, because to Love the Heavenly Father means Loving One Another!

Also, Love your Mother in Nature as She Loves you, because it was She who created, nursed, taught you to walk your first steps and gave you all that you are. Love, also, all of Humanity, without regard to color of skin, or to what nation they belong, because this means Loving God and Nature.

The Wisdom of all this shall be seen when all of Mankind on earth learns to Love one another just as God Loves each and everyone of us; Heaven will be realized on earth since it will cease to be a Vale of Tears and turn into a Valley of Happiness and great Joy of Living. Then shall all hatred, all evil, fighting and wars cease, and Peace will prevail thru Good Will among Mankind. Each individual shall show and feel this Good Will by keeping the Law of Love, seeking to comfort one another, their neighbors, their friends and even more, their enemies. They shall seek to please them, to serve them without self interest, so that this earth may become a radiant star of Love.

When mankind becomes Spiritualized, Divine Gifts shall be found common among humans, because with this discipline of behavior, certain endocrine secretion glands which are latent but undeveloped in the human body as yet and await activation, shall be awakened thru the soul becoming mature enough to make use of them. Such is the case with Astral Vision which enables one to see even those who have left their bodies and visit with them. Becoming more advanced they shall become free and able to get acquainted with the metaphysical or higher planes, living in this world and in the world's beyond this one. Once humans become spiritually evolved enough, they shall not need to reincarnate again and again on earth, having learned all that earth living affords. Their perfection shall be continued on planes more advanced than the physical in what is called Heaven. Joyously our Heavenly Father shall receive them as a part of Heaven, and they shall inherit or share Supreme Being in the Infinity of Cosmos. By Love the Heavenly Father creates His Sons and Daughters, by Love He teaches and prepares them for the Higher Life in His Heavenly Realm. By Love the Heavenly Father creates His Sons and Daughters, by Love He teaches and prepares them for the Higher Life in His Heavenly Realm. By Love He shall receive us in His Heavenly Kingdom, and by Love we shall participate in Everlasting Life, Happiness and Glory.

Love is the motive power that moves all the Universe. Love is the most powerful and safest means of power that never fails because it is the only one that is Eternal and in perpetual motion. To give you a fuller view of this Life, I have given you a faint glimpse of what lays beyond. Undoubtedly this still remains somewhat a mystery to you which you shall only understand as time goes on. Meanwhile you only need Faith, great Faith, and to believe in my Word, because I speak the Word of my Heavenly Father, and only the Word of Truth, the Gnosis shall flow from my lips.

So, in Truth I tell you, when you get to know the Presence of your Heavenly Father within you, the veil shall be lifted from your vision, and you shall know both the Mysteries of Life on earth and in the Heavens. Then you shall no longer need Faith, which will be replaced with the Gnosis (Divine Knowledge of Truth), without the need to blindly believe or put Faith in anything.

Ed. Notes: "All are but a part of one stupendous whole,
    Whose body Nature is, and God the Soul."

CHAPTER XII (1-21)

However, I do realize that a great part of my teachings are Mysteries that seem a riddle to you. The reason you do not understand them is because you have sought Wisdom in books, Scriptures of a Dead Word in a dead tongue. They were written by dead men in spirit as well as body, and they are now also interpreted and explained by men who are the living dead whose souls dwell in unclean, intoxicated bodies, dead to true Life, materialists without the slightest bit of Spiritual Vision. Thus, it is easy for you to understand their teaching because you also dwell in diseased bodies filled with impurities, which prevent Spiritual Insight, like a dark cloud prevents one from seeing the Sun. It follows that you see everything wrong, so you know not the Truth. You are guided by the blind, following blindly, which is the very reason you are suffering sickness in pain, and without Faith, walk in sin. To remove you from this disaster, the Heavenly Father sent me to make the Light of Life shine within you, which is the Light of the Gnosis of my Faith, Hope and Truth.

In the meantime, you were not prepared to bear such Illumination because your vision is used to Darkness only, so you cannot bear the intense Light of the Heavenly Father. To understand this teaching, I sent my Angels to prepare your understanding to be able to get Insight without being blinded or flinching. With the kind aid of Nature's Angels, the Angels of Sunshine, Air, Water, Fasting, Enemas and others, your bodies will become strengthened and become sensitive so as to be able to understand my Transcendent Teaching of Truth, the Gnosis.

Also, you shall be able to gaze at the mid-day sun without flinching. However, at first you must be very careful because if you do not, you may damage your vision or become blind. At first look at the early morning sun after sunrise, or when it sets. At other times just look at it for an instant, opening and closing your eyes. When your body becomes perfectly clean and purified within, your eyes will be able to bear more and more sunlight without being blinded. Thus, will you also be able to bear a more intense Light, even to see the Heavenly Father face to face, whose Light is infinitely greater than hundreds of suns.

Without a thorough, cleansing of your bodies, both the physical and spiritual bodies, or body and soul, you should not seek to contemplate the sun because it may provoke visual disorders. If you believe I am sent by the Father in the Heavens, and have Faith in my teachings, along with the practical application of the blessings of Nature which I described as Angels, you shall be ever free from disease and pain, and thus enjoy perfect health, peace, Happiness and Long Life. The Heavenly Father loves those who forsake their evil ways and follow Him, seeking Him in prayer, letting Him show them the solution to their problems. They shall be blessed with the good things of Life, rewarding their Faith in the Universal Father. For what is impossible for men, is quite possible and only a trifle for Almighty God, so He surely can solve your problems. To restore your health, He sends you His Divine Messengers, His Angels, to serve and guide you along the Path of Right Living.

May you Live in Love which is the Light of God.

CHAPTER XIII (1-16)

During the day, the Savior taught the multitudes that crowded around him because they all wanted to be close to Him, and to receive the Emanations of Divine Power, Peace and Happiness of his resplendent aura. After nightfall, the moon appeared among the fleeing clouds as its silvery rays illumined the face of our Lord.

Suddenly, the Anointed of Spirit stood up and to the amazement of all those present, he was transfigured. He shone like the sun as He arose above the earth heavenward. No one dared to move or say a word, for they were held motionless in awe, dumbfoundly gazing at this magnificent appearance of the Anointed. Time stood still so no one knew how much time passed. Opening up His arms extended in a spiritual embrace He bid them farewell, saying "Peace be with you"! Immediately He was hidden among the clouds before their very eyes. Speechless, they remained as if in a deep sleep.

The next day at dawn they awoke marvelling about their heavenly dreams whose witness strengthened their Faith in Christ. It was a wonderful awakening: Heavenly music, soft and sweet penetrated their surroundings and they were filled with indescribable happiness. But at last one said to another, "What a wonderful night,- if only it could be everlasting". Others remarked, "What a Joy to have been here". Still others, "In truth he is one sent by God, because only he is able to give us lasting peace, fill us with happiness and give us hope for better times."

Following this magnificent experience of dawn, came a radiant sunrise with warming rays inviting them to enjoy a sunbath, for now they were convinced at heart that the Sun was their star of hope for the wonderful future new world and age to come,- a world of Peace, Understanding, Justice and Love. Thus, all of them, together contentedly and happily began walking to a nearby stream of crystal clear, pure water which seemed to be beckoning them to partake of its waters. There they found the Angels of the Lord waiting for them to come cleanse their bodies that splendid morning.

=:=:=:=:=:=:=

Editor's Notes concerning Luminous appearances of the Savior among the Apostles and Spiritual Kingdom of Light within us:- From "The Gnostic Religion" by Hans Jonas we quote from scattered parts of the book: "Of inestimable value for the knowledge of Gnosticism are the Sacred Books of the Mandaeans, no less violently anti-Christian than anti-Jewish, but including among its prophets John the Baptist, in opposition to, and at the expense of Christ. They felt violently hostile to Christian Doctrine, whose Founder, according to Mandaean tradition had stolen and falsified the message of his Master

(John). The name (Mandaean) is derived from Aramaic MANDA, "knowledge" so that Mandaeans are literally Gnostics. The Mandaean "Mana"...is the name for the transmundane Power of LIGHT, the First Deity, Highest Godhead and at the same time that for the transcendent nonmundane center of individual ego. Manda d'Hayye was the Knowledge of Life, the Gnosis personified in the central Divine Savior figure of Mandaean Religion, called forth by the Life in the worlds of Light, and sent down to the lower worlds. Manda d'Hayye revealed himself to man to redeem him from darkness to Light. Flowing water Mandaeans called "Jordans"...an indication of geographic origin of Mandaean communities...they only settled close to rivers. In a Mandaean text Urtha of Life spoke: "Be silent Adam, thou head of the whole tribe. The world which is to be we cannot suppress. Arise, worship the Great Life and submit thyself that Life may be thy Savior. The Life be thy Savior and do thou ascend and behold the place of Light." "From the point of view of the history of Religion, Manichaeism is the most important product of Gnosticism." In conclusion, Hans Jonas' viewpoint is of vital importance when he says, "Mani had the only Gnostic System of historic force that must be ranked among the major religions of mankind."

Mani was born in the Parthian kingdom on the 14th of April, 216 A.D. of Persian parents. His father was of the John Baptist sect of Mandaeans and he was educated in a school of Mandaean Religion, so that his writings show an influence of the Mandaean models. Yet Mani's catholicity went far beyond what now passes as the Catholic or Christian Churches, for this was truly the FIRST ATTEMPT to establish the true UNIVERSAL RELIGION and model for the Heavenly Ecclesia. His main activity was under Shapur (214-272) and he was crucified under Bahram I (277). It was the threat of this new Universal Religion in world power that a generation after Mani the so-called Catholic or Universal Church in Rome was organized under the leadership of Saint Constantine (Nicea, 325) seeking to ignore and prevent Gnostic religious influence, in Persia, from overwhelming the ailing Roman empire. Rome had true primitive Christians exiled to the East or killed.

Mani's father heard a voice that commanded him to abstain from meat, wine and sexual relations, repeatedly, which led him to join a John Baptist Gnostic community to practice his beliefs, where Mani was born. With such spiritual aid from birth (miraculously as told of in N.T. allegories), Mani also had two outstanding visits of the Holy Spirit, one at 12 and another at 24. His writings also show he received the teachings of the Gnostic St. Thomas concerning the "Double", "Twin" of our Lord in Spiritual significance, being one thru the Communion of Saints, as taught early First Christians, preparing him to preach the gospel. This explains the fact Mani spent 2 years almost receiving indoctrination in India, realizing Buddhist truths. According to a Compendium of Doctrines of Mani,- the Buddha of Light,- his affirmed teachings consisted of: (1) A Universal Religion, (2) of Eternal Foundation thru the ages, (3) to save souls who have not obtained salvation in present beliefs, (4) the Revelation of his Books of Life, Wisdom and Gnosis being beyond the scope of past religions.

Mani wrote his Books of Life because (1) Mani is wherever his books are read, (2) disciples have a duty to translate them so others may know his truths, (3) having been put into writing, there is no room for arguing about principles as with prior doctrines. Here was the first attempt in recorded history to deliberately take the most important and most universal concepts of Buddhism, Zoroastrianism and Primitive Gnostic Christianity to form a truly Ecumenical, Catholic or Universal Religion. He held that God had nothing evil with which to punish matter. Our desires are not for being, but for possessing the better, and its recognition is not one of love but of resentment. "The Father of Greatness called forth the Mother of Life, and the Mother of Life called forth Primal Man", so this Primal Man (Adam) was the emanation of the Highest Godhead. (All this shows identity to our Johannine teaching of Healing God Spell above). The Light within is Changeless, Eternal and Immutable.

Mani wrote (Shahpuraken): "From aeon to aeon, the Apostles of God did not cease to bring here Wisdom and the Works. Thus, in one age the coming was into the land of India thru the Apostle known as the Buddha; in another age into the land of Persia thru Zoroaster; in another to the land in the West thru a "Jesus." After that, in the last age, this revelation came down and this prophethood arrived thru myself, Mani, the Apostle of the true God in the land of Babylonia." Thus, like the Aramaic "Mana" being the Godhead in Light, so "Mani" indicates the Son of the Godhead in Gnostic terminology and history.

This Godhead is the Luminous Self or Savior, so when Mani spoke of Jesus he would show this meaning: "Jesus the Luminous approached Adam and awakened him from the sleep of death", just as with Buddha, Zoroaster and others before Mani, all of whom received the original Light of Gnosis thru the Luminous Savior who existed since the foundation of the world and universe. Mani's doctrine included the doctrine of "Jesus patibilis", "who hangs from every tree, is served up in every dish, everyday is born, suffers and dies." He is dispersed in all Creation, but his most genuine realm and embodiment seems to be in the vegetable world, the most passive and only innocent form of life. "One should abstain from all ensouled things and eat only vegetables and whatever else is non-sentient, and abstain from marriage, the delights of love and begetting children to free Divine Power from successive generations of suffering on earth." Also like the Buddha, Mani taught against building, made the people aware of destroying Life when they walked on grass or tread on tiny animal life on the ground, beside disciples needing to abstain from all types of animal food including milk and eggs. Against the haunting appeal people have for ceremony and myth, he preached the ceremony of daily life, which is hidden in the mysteries that religions pretend to practice in their rituals. The clasping of right hands dates back to the Manichaeans, still in practice even among the Churches opposing the original Gnostic Christians, the N.T. Bible commanding the "Kiss of Peace" which betrayed their Savior, and back in the 1940s in Catholic Ecuador the fraternal embrace was preferred to the "Capitalist" handshake, altho the origins were known, not disclosed. With the change of times, Gnostics are using the embrace and Catholics the handclasp! Mani's doctrine and their communities spread from Persia to Egypt beside east to China. In the Gobi desert, the fabled region of "Shamballa" Sacred Island, and a short distance from one of my teacher's dominions (Pr. Cherenzi Lind, Ch'An Cheng Lob, Tihwa of Chinese Turkistan) at the oasis Turfan, Manichaean archives tell about the Living Luminous Self in all, "Mana", etc. It also reveal the source of the Spiritual Hierarchies of the Tibetan Gobi mysticism such as the Great White Brotherhood and Lodge of Theosophists and related doctrines, which are absent from Southern Buddhist beliefs. Gnostic Christians are known to have arrived in the Gobi, Tibet and China in the first three centuries before the founding of Rome's Catholicism in the 4th century, and the arrival of Buddhism in 7th century Tibet.

However the most sensational find was revealed in the 1945 discovery of Nag Hammadi, ancient Chenoboskion Library in Upper Egypt, which are to be published completely now, which with mentioned Turfan manuscripts, beside others at Fayum of Egypt and the famous Dead Sea Scrolls, should reveal the true nature of the Gnostic origins of both Christian and Buddhist Apostolic Hierarchies and beliefs. The Chenoboskion Sacred Library is predominant in Sethian books showing the community to be Sethian. In "Revelations of Adam to his Son Seth" there is the original doctrine of Succession of 13 Enlighteners (Christs, Buddhas, aeons or Avatars) coming down into the world, each giving a fuller Gnosis.

In "The Gnostic Religion" Jonas writes, "There would then be some kind of continuity between the disappearing Essene movement and the emerging Sethian Gnosis," explains Doressi's suggestion that since Gomorrah and Sodom are ancient Essene colonies, and Seth took his seed in Gomorrah, which is believed to be Qumran (of Dead Sea Scroll fame) and sowed it in Sodom after Qumran was destroyed, since Sodom is said to be the dwelling place of Great Seth. Thus, thru the Illumined Gnostics, or Angel-Savior, from Seth,- whose tribe smelled like the trees of Paradise and nourished exclusively from fruits, Buddha who lived from forest food before Sambodhi, John the Baptist who ate no meat, bread or anything but wild carob fruit and nectars, Mani who also ate no animal product, and others, I have received the Gnosis of my past Incarnations for the New Age and Race Salvation Message of Love-Wisdom. No one in history, or legend even, has taught why and how bloodshed can be completely eliminated, not only in the killing of men and animals, but women's monthly bleeding including ovulation and seminal losses in men which deny purity with fetid odors, beside the benefits of the complete integrity of valuable body substances and avoiding pathological microorganism production. The Sethians claimed generative powers were the Beast or Serpent, due to the hissing sound the female organ makes and the shape of the male organ, but the pure and virgin womb was believed to be able to produce immortal humans thru the Spheres of Light. This is the descent of Perfect Man, Mana or Logos, which will destroy the birth pangs of carnal man. This same practice is used combined with Buddhist Philosophy in the Mahayana theory of forming the Divine Body, Dharma Kaya of Truth Light which stops attachment to the wheel of births and deaths in the world of suffering and in compassion saving humanity by example. With the realization of the Divine Body of Light and Truth, identifying Self outside the body and on the Inner planes is the escape from mortality, so one can transfer consciousness from body to body, even materialize bodies out of thin air, and live thousands of years without death receiving fresh new body vehicles from volunteers who by initiation give up theirs for Mastery. Vitalogy will bring the Dharma Kaya and the Gnostic Virgin Conception of the Light Body to the practical Paradisian Living Powers of the New Race thru Regenerative Sublimation and Transmutation of one's mortal physical body. These were the prophetic implications hidden in the N.T. allegories on Eternal Life and Life in the Resurrection, One in the Body and Light of Christ, Luminous Savior.

The teaching of the Jordan as the source of cleansing water of Baptism, and on the other hand, the teaching of sexual transmutation or making the Jordan flow back to its Source, actually made for the breaking among two extremes, those following Simon Peter as the cornerstone of the Church of Rome, and the Disciple of John. Marcion, still remembered as the "Most Christian" of Gnostics, made an attack on the Baptism of John when it became ritualized:- "The river Jordan is the strength of the body, the essence of pleasures, and the water of the Jordan is the desire for Carnal cohabitation. John himself is the Archon of the multitude!" Underlying all these heated debates of Gnostics, are seen the basic tenets of Buddhist missionaries combined with Tantric Kundalini Yoga.

Just as Savior (Jesus) and John are identical persons, both being born of the same father, Zacharias, in the same year, with the same stories of Immaculate Conception by the Holy Spirit, seen by comparing the Protevangelion and Luke I N.T. stories, are baptised in the Jordan, and are seen in resurrections and miracles, so the wise will know John was the body born of woman whose Divine Body by living on wild fruits, carob and nectars (wild honey), the Living Water of Everlasting Life. However, the Simon "Pure" doctrine which Rome took, came because eating grains, Christians like Buddhists, were so sexually stimulated that they needed to sublimate artificially what came naturally by John's way.

CHAPTER XIV (1-20)

All those among them of one accord came together on the brook's shore with clear waters that came splashing down from higher regions finally forming a delightful shower at the waterfall. Also, the news that the Savior was preaching there brought many people from their vicinity as well as from afar seeking that the Healer might heal them.

The Anointed of Spirit spoke with them and taught them, inviting them to take off their sandals and clothing, and to partake of the beneficial action provided by the Angels of Sunshine, Air and Water while they fasted their bodies. One by one, they all partook of the refreshing shower, baptizing them in the waters that noisily fell from above, followed by rolling on the warm sand, in contact with earth, sunbathing.

In this way the Angels of Mother Nature began in them a wonderful work of purification, hygiene and strengthening of their weak and sickly bodies. All these sick people were amazed to see how they could eliminate such great amounts of filth from their bodies, feeling an agreeable wonder of surprise about it, as well as the pain and symptoms of elimination tormenting to bear. Some of them had a nauseating foul breath that smelled like a rotting carcass that they could hardly bear themselves. Others vomited great amounts and suffered diarrheas of unbearable stench. The wonderful effects of these Angels of Purification became more intense with time, so that some of the patients had eliminations thru their noses, their ears, their eyes, and their throats in cases relieving them of persistent headaches which had long tormented them. Many perspired profusely thru their skin eliminating a sweat that smelled so bad that those around them had to remove to a distance. Many developed festering skin sores that turned into ulcers expelling a smelly pus with blood; others had urine with pus or with blood, as well as containing grit and stones from within. Some also belched forth evil-smelling gases from their mouths and their bowels.

Their internal baths also began to produce amazing results. They prepared enemas with clear, clean water from the brook warmed in the sun. They held this water in their bowels, which came with abominable soft or hard matter of an unbearable smell, matter that had adhered to the intestinal walls for many years infecting the blood of the patients as well as their whole organism, being the very cause of their many infectious diseases, unbearable aches and tormenting ailments. In the water that gushed out from their bowels were to be found horrible worms of all sizes, some very long, which writhed in the hot sunshine. Many of them trembled with horror to see such terrible abominations that they had eliminated from their own bowels. But now their insides, becoming clean, no longer had fever and pain, and they clearly understood why these repulsive abominations were the precise cause of their chronic illness. They rendered thanks to the Lord for having sent the kind Angels who had driven out the devils from their bowels causing their torment. Nevertheless, not all were freed from their pains. These disillusioned few went in search of the Master to complain about their suffering, so that thru his power he might remove the stubborn and possessive demons who refused to depart from them.

=:=:=:=:=:=

EDITOR'S NOTES (continued from the last Chapter).

THE MYSTICAL SPHERES OF LIGHT WITHIN	LOCATION	KUNDALINI CHAKRA
7. Mt. Hermon, Holy Mt. of Transfiguration (Meru)	headtop	Sahasrara
6. Caesarea Philippi, Road to Damascus vision	forehead	Agna
5. Lake Huleh, Mermon, clairaudience	throat	Vishudha
4. Sea of Galilee, Cana, Nazareth, mastery	heart	Anahata
3. Jacob's Well, Living Water, Eternal Life	solar plexus	Manipuri
2. Bethany, Transjordan, Regeneration	sex organs	Swadhisthana
1. Mouth of Jordan, Spiritual re-direction	perineum	Muladhara

To realize the Spheres of Light of the Great Body of the Heavenly Man, within, or enter the Ogdoad giving Immortality, one must turn back the Mystic Jordan River, preventing entry into the Dead Sea, for which the N.T. allegories taking place in the named Mystical Spheres regions of Palestine are studied to learn the Powers and Mastery which are acquired by prayer, continence and living water baptisms. Life Swirls, Vortices or Light Spheres of Gnostic symbols correspond to Yoga Mystical Chakras, as do Sacred River locations.

CHAPTER XV (1-68) THE HEALING GOD SPELL OF SAINT JOHN

When they went to search for the Master, he already knew they urgently needed him and was immediately found approaching where they were, causing them to marvel and rejoice when he greeted them, "Peace be unto you!" The Anointed of Spirit added, "Yes, I know why you seek me! You seek me now because you want me to heal you when you are in intense pain, and suffering so much that nothing else can enter your mind!" He then explained to them a parable that left them in even greater astonishment, realizing how well he knew all their needs and could speak with such Wisdom: "You are like the PRODIGAL SON who for many years abused the patience of his Father. He neglected his sacred obligation in his duties by shunning his responsibilities in work, preferring to spend his time enjoying himself in festivity and pleasure-seeking with his friends, eating and drinking at his father's expense. Without his father's knowledge, he continued to incur new debts spending all his father's money he could get his hands upon, which he squandered in the company of his friends. The moneylenders willingly always lent him more money, knowing that his father was wealthy and always would with patience willingly cancel his son's debts. In vain his father spoke to him, asking him to shape up his character with kindly and persuasive words, admonishing his son, who, in turn, always continued to say he would do better, but instead of behaving, he continued to behave worse.

Uselessly, his father would always tell him to stop his riotous excess and corrupt living, and to come help him in the work he needed done in the fields, overseeing the workers in their labor. Yet, always the son would promise to amend his ways so that his father would again pay up the son's most recent loans. Then again, his son would continue in his vicious ways of life, promising always to correct his ways and make right what he owed his father. Thus, for seven years his son continued to abuse his father. There then came a time when his father's patience came to an abrupt end. He refused to pay the Usurers. He now told the moneylenders that if he continued to pay them continually, he not only lost all he gave them, but his son was lost with it all. If he refused to pay, he had only both to gain from it! Now, the usurers, seeing they were out of their money, lost all hope of being paid. They took the son to the Judge, who in turn gave the son to the moneylenders as a slave, that he might pay back what he had squandered by his own work to pay off the debt. This was according to the severity of the Law and the custom in those days.

This certainly put an end to the licentious life of the son. From dawn to dusk he worked, now obliged to do very heavy work digging up the ground, to cultivate it, to plant it and to harvest the crops. For the first time in his life he now earned his bread with the sweat of his brow. Since he was not accustomed to this hard work, his muscles in the arms ached and withered. His hands and feet became covered with blisters. For the first time in his life he knew what hunger was, for now he only had bread with water to eat and drink. In the seventh day of such hard work, he said to his new master to whom he had become enslaved, "No longer can I endure such heavy labor. I am not used to it. Look, my hands are all blisters, unable to do work, and my feet also are so tender I cannot walk. All my strength at length has left me. My body has become skin and bones. Have mercy on me. Why make me suffer anymore?" But the slave master answered him sternly without paying any attention to his suffering: "Only when you have completed the seven years of work you owe me so as to cancel the debt you created, will you be free. Now, get back to your work!"

The desperate laborer then cried out: "But I have suffered all I possible can these past seven days. I am about to faint, worn out with no more strength to go on this way working at such unaccustomed labor. Have compassion on me. My hands are bleeding from the blisters and my feet are so swollen that I no longer am able to walk or work." However the cruel creditor only hurried him on in his work ruthlessly: "If you could waste away your days and nights for seven years in pleasures you enjoyed without limits accumulating such a great debt with me, certainly now you must be able to pay back that debt with seven years of work. I will not forgive you till you pay the uttermost drachma. Now, the slave master threatened him giving him a lashing of his whip, so he could no longer refuse to obey and was forced to continue working. After his day's work, the prodigal son could endure no more. He gathered together his last bit of strength, and managed to get to his father's house. He threw himself before his father's feet, begging of him, "Father, believe me for this last time now it is the last time I will ever offend you. I swear that never again will I return to my life of unrestrained pleasure seeking, and now I shall become a model son. I see my error and shall correct the injustice. Father, free me of my oppressors. But now even his own father said nothing. Now, he too distrusted such a liar. After he had been only abused every time he believed his son in so many promises, he could only distrust him with severity. So again his son kept insisting as he wept, saying:

"Father, be not hardened of heart, look at my bleeding blistered hands, that have come from working with a mattock, the scythe and the sickle. See how my feet are swollen and blistered. Have mercy on me for I truly repent all I did."

This time, the sincere pleading softened his father's heart. Now, with tears of happiness flowing from his eyes he took his son in his arms, saying: "Let us rejoice together, because you have this day given me joy. I have finally found my long lost son! He again clothed his son in choice raiment, and they finished the day celebrating the reunion merrily. The next day, the father gave his son a bag of money with which to cancel the debts he had with his creditors, so as to be freed from further obligation to serve them as a slave. Returning from this, his father said, "You see, my son, how easy it is to accumulate such a great debt thru a life of lust and dishonesty. How hard it is to pay back this debt thru your own effort with labor when forced to do so.

"Father, how true that is, I now know, because not even for only seven days can I endure it!" "Beloved son, this one and last time I have allowed you to pay your debts in seven days only. All the rest shall be forgiven thee if you forever abandon your life of seeking pleasures and henceforth no longer acquire debts, as the condition of this grant.

The Heavenly Teacher continued explaining, "Truly, truly I say unto you, only the Father, and no one else is able to forgive the sins of his children, and this is true only when they sincerely repent and are really sorry they have sinned. They must not only ask for forgiveness, but also do penance with constraint in their hearts, and firmly determine in will not to backslide again into evil paths.

Now likewise, the father said, "My son, had I not pardoned your sin this time, you know you would have been obliged to repay your debts with seven years of slavery this being our Law. His son replied, My Father, from the depth of my heart I thank thee, and from now on I promise always to be your worthy son, an example of one who respects his responsibilities keeping your commandments. Never again will I run up debts for you on my account now that I have experienced how hard it is to repay them." His son did just as he had promised: He forsook his sinful way of life and became a dedicated worker, wholeheartedly helping his father watching over his Father's work in the field, helping in what ever he could do. Then the Father saw how well he complied with his promises, and as the years passed, the land dedicated to his Father's work increased under his hand. Finally, his father willed all his wealth of land, tools, houses, and beasts of burden to this worthy son. In turn his son, when he became the lord of all his father possessed, he busied himself making sure that when there were some who owed debts they could not pay, their debts he would also pardon, thus, ever remembering how hard it had been for him to pay his with hard labor."

"In our lives, what is true first with our carnal father, is also true in regard to our Heavenly Father, who shall bless the worthy son's and daughters with long life, good health, a faithful soul mate, many spiritual sons and daughters, good fortune, enjoying everlasting peace and happiness to an advanced age. All this shall come true by truly regenerating our own lives, and then justly dealing with all our brothers and sisters among humanity, all the animals, the birds of the skies and all who are subject to our Heavenly Father and Mother Nature.

Editor's Note: St. John, the Initiator, used the shock method of illustrating and teaching in his method, as do modern Vajrayana Buddhist Teachers. Whether we realize it or not, the Adversities, and the severe Crisis in our lives are Spiritual or Mystical Initiations, just as in the prodigal son's slave epoch.

CHAPTER XVI (1-16)

Then the Anointed Savior turned to the other sick patients and said: "I speak to you in PARABLES because it makes God's Word and Commandments clearer to understand. The seven years of eating, drinking and riotous living are one's past sins against God's Commandments, which include the inviolable obligation to obey the Laws of Natural Living, symbolized by the Angels of Sunshine, Air, Water, Fasting, Enemas, Rational Living, Prayer, etc. The cruel creditor or usurer is symbolized by a wicked Satan, which is really a non-existent fictional character, because it represents our own evil habits, our vices and our sins: What he really amounts to is our IGNORANCE, because those who are wise will keep the Lord's Commandments, and are NEVER SICK NOR SUFFER PAIN.

The debts are the disease one acquires, because of one's Ignorance which made one disobey the Laws of Natural Living. The hard labor represents the aches and pains one has to suffer, which are harder to endure than the effort one has to make to work. The prodigal son is yourselves in your violation of the Heavenly Father's Commandments which are the Natural Laws of this Life. The payment of debts acquired against one's moral obligations, consists of elimination of one's vices and evil habits from one's character, purifying one's soul, because this is what will take away one's disease and pains one has to suffer. THIS IS TRUE, BECAUSE ONLY THE LIVING SOUL SINS, SINCE THE BODY, WHICH IS INERT MATTER (like a dead corpse) OF ITSELF CANNOT SIN. The bag of silver received from the Father symbolizes paying the reward required for one's release or freedom, which will make possible robust health and a long life thru Regeneration and a return to the Path of Living Righteously. The Father is none other than the Author of all that is, God of the Heavens and the Universe. His servants are Holy Angels which symbolize the means by which one may purify oneself to get in closer and closer contact with the Heavenly Father, such as the Sunshine, Air, Water, Fasting, Virtuous Living, Prayer, etc. until one finally identifies with God himself.

The possessions belonging to our Father are the whole Universe: the Heavens, the sun, the earth, the stars and the planets, so that there is enough space for all of God's children. All of this whole Universe is the field of the Father, his lands, his crops and wherever the children of Mankind may collaborate harmoniously in the works of the Heavenly Father, which is all of Creation, so as to be worthy of reward and good fortune, if they will first humbly keep the Natural Laws here on earth.

Now, my beloved ones, I ask you, is it not more sensible and reasonable to obey our Father, helping him in his work, earning our daily food by honest labor, rather than worthless merry-making, as a spender who requires money, and spending excessively to the wicked creditors (or bankers) who exploit one unjustly, so that when it comes time to pay our debts, one has to work seven years as a slave? Likewise, is it not wiser, also, to obey God, working in harmony with Nature, or His Creation, enjoying the good fortune of having good health, a long life filled with joy and happiness, rather than disobeying our Father, so as to live in misery, pain, unwanted, sick ailing, bitter, depressed and unhappy with life? Remember that by your behavior you yourselves are who determine or carve out your own destiny, whether you live happy or unhappy, healthy or unhealthy, with good or evil fortune, because as you sow, so shall you reap!

CHAPTER XVII (1-11)

The number of sins and offences that you have committed against Mother Nature is certainly very great and of many kinds, I assure you. For years you have sinned in shameful pleasures against moral decency by which I mean against the Natural Laws of Life. You have not lived according to these Laws by enjoying yourselves by overeating, drunkenness, fornication, and so many other vices too many to name even. In this way, you have defiled your soul and poisoned your body, until you have hardly anything but a stinking corpse to live with, due to all these diseases that you have brought on with your evil behavior (Karma).

Now, you have to suffer the consequences of your errors, your sins committed against Mother Nature. However, do not despair, because also great is the Mercy of our Heavenly Father, even toward his wasteful, pleasure-seeking children, if they will repent and return to Him to ask Forgiveness, for He shall forgive the offences you have committed. Remember, that great and infinite is the Love of our Heavenly Father for all his penitent followers who ask for forgiveness. Our Heavenly Father is so moved by our humble submission, our prayer and our repentance when we return to the Presence of God that He will accept the payment of the debt in seven days what otherwise required seven years of forced labor in slavery, if one will sincerely repent asking forgiveness of our all-seeing Heavenly Father.

"But, what if one has sinned seven times seven years,- will the Lord forgive us then?" asked a sick old man. "Exactly, even in such cases, if they sincerely repent their sins, our Heavenly Father shall forgive those who have sinned seven times seven years, by reducing their suffering to having to fast only seven times these seven days repeatedly."

CHAPTER XVIII (1-11)

Whosoever shall persevere to the end in their Path of Perfection, they shall live in Bliss. Whosoever shall with a firm pace and determined resolve cross the finish line or goal shall be worthy of laurels of victory. All the triumphs and downfalls that you encounter in life's laborious career, all our virtues and errors, are recorded in NATURE'S MEMORY in an eternal indelible memorandum of all our past lives. For they are written in your own bodies and souls, which are like an open book exposed to God's vision, and in astonishing faithfulness tell the whole history of our past lives. Even your most secret thoughts are written naturally and subconsciously in this Eternal Memorandum, where they remain recorded from the beginning of time to eternity. So that when you come before your Heavenly Father, which inevitable happens right here where we are living on earth, His trained vision will at once read the history of your behavior, rejoicing in your good works and saddened when you fall short, committing evil actions. So perfect is this genetic record in your Book of Life that there is not the slightest detail that escapes its accuracy. You may often escape justice according to man-made laws, but Divine Justice, never.

However, if you repent your sins soon enough, and seek out the kind servants or elements of Nature, which are the Guiding Angels of Mother Nature as found in Sunshine, Air, Water, Fasting, Prayer, etc.. and if you practice all the great virtues known to mankind based on Love, then these scars and defects shall be removed from your body and soul so that the good signs remain recorded in your Living Book. When you have removed every page recording the evil accounts, and you again have a clean Genetic Memory, free of all defects disfavorable to your body then you shall again be worthy of the Heavenly Presence of God. Likewise the Heavenly Father's heart shall rejoice to see that his prodigal son or daughter, has returned penitent and willing to serve his parental home. He shall receive you with honor and rejoice to read in your Living Book of Life, how you have triumphed thru all obstacles and difficulties that prevented you from access in getting up to a Cosmic Abode, and how you succeeded in removing all the sins from that great book. Then shall the Heavenly Father reward your efforts, granting you long life on earth, without sickness and pain, without ailments and suffering, beside serene peace and everlasting happiness. You will meet with good fortune in everything you do. God will send forth Angels from Heaven and his Servants in Nature to guide you into the best of everything and guard you from evil paths. If from this moment onward you dedicate yourself to selfless service of humanity, doing good to others then shall the Highest raise you up into the Highest Positions in His HEAVENLY

HIERARCHY as a Co-worker, with special gifts and powers. And when you leave this plane on this planet, you shall ascend even higher into the Father's Kingdom of Heaven beyond earth in the hereafter where there shall be Everlasting Life and Happiness. Fortunate indeed are they whosoever with driving perseverance and tenacious effort conquer the worthiness to be able to enter the Kingdom of Heaven, for there shall be no more suffering, no sickness, nor pain, nor old age, nor death, but instead perfect health, perfect joy in living in Eternity. (Removing self from the wheel of births and deaths we reach NIRVANA).

CHAPTER XIX (1-30)

Immediately, leaving the multitude he bid them farewell with his blessing with arms outstretched saying, "Peace be with you!" Then he hastened to a group of invalids who lay helpless on the ground, unable to do anymore than crawl with great effort. They cried out, "Oh Master, Master have mercy on us in our deformities and suffering. What can we do to heal ourselves from our disabilities and pain?" Some showed him their swollen and aching feet, others with knotted or twisted bones out of joint; still others had ulcers, sores and other skin inflammations, which showed their internal uncleanliness with external eruptions. The Divinely Anointed, filled with compassion, sought to inspire them with courage by assuring them that, with all certainty, your ailments shall be healed, if you shall endure fasting for more than the seven days, since the seriousness of your chronic ailments came about with grievous violations. Do not despair, have faith. Behold, I shall offer another angel to help you, the ANGEL OF EARTH!" He pointed his hand to a swampy, muddy flat, consisting of soft clay or mud. "Now, bury your naked bodies in this mud, leaving only your heads out, and patiently and faithfully await the healing action of this marvellous Angel of Earth, and the powerful Angel of Sunshine which will heat or warm the muddy clay and charge it with solar energy."

Those who were ailing did that very thing. Many of them immediately were relieved, pleased actually, upon being buried in this soft, warm and attracting substance that at once drew out the pain and fever within that so often affected their stomach, intestines and well being. And so, fasting and praying, buried for days at a length in this healing mud bath, listening to the consoling words of the Divine Physician which were more nourishing than food to them, a Spiritual Food, they endured. Also, there were others who shouted, "Master, I am healed of ailments that we suffered for many years!" Others, in great joy, told how their swollen members had reduced or completely healed, being relieved of chronic pains that they had endured for years. Still others rejoiced calling out that their bones had returned to their former natural position, rather than twisted, so they could walk erect and effortlessly. To show what had happened they came out of their mud bath, and feebly managed to walk over to the Master. Finally, even others whose skin had been troubled with ulcers, sores, or other inflammations, since their first day in the mud had experienced notable relief, their skin healed from defects, and after several days they now showed, a skin smooth and vigorous for others to see as they proclaimed it to all.

Their Instructor then commanded those who had left their mud baths healed to take a shower under the crystalline waterfall that fell from a spring located far above which fell like a heavy downpour of rain. Rapidly they washed off every bit of mud, and exhibited their healed and vigorous new appearance. After observing attentively the condition of each patient, he instructed them to dry their bodies lying on the warm sand on the shore rolling over on front and back. This they enjoyed doing spending sometime in this dry warm sand heated by the sun. When completely dry, they again rejoiced as they gave thanks to their Divine Healer. With sincere emotion they all prostrated and kissed his feet in thanks for these wonders of healing. All the thousands who had gathered there, from the most humble to the highest chief officials of Government, Pharisees, Scribes and Priests, all of them, some with envy, and others well pleased, were able to witness these miraculous healings realized under the direction of the Master Healer.

The last one to leave the mud bath was a young man, who his brothers brought dragging on his cot, because he had lost consciousness and his skin had turned blackish; His brothers said that this came about due to a snake bite of a poisonous species. So, instead of dismissing him, the Savior instructed them to bury him again in the mud, keeping watch over him till he regained consciousness and was again perfectly healthy. Consequently, following the instructions caring for this man, he too was healed, and all were astonished to see how the once-blackish skin now glowed, filled with a rosy color, after he recovered consciousness and was restored in health. After he got dry in the warm sand, he too came and fell down to bathe the Divine Master's feet with tears of happiness, as did also his brethren. The Savior, visibly moved then said, "Do not give thanks to me, but instead, to my Father, who sent me to heal your ailments. Now, return to your respective communities and proclaim to all the healing effects and benefits of the Angel-Messengers of Sunshine, Air, Water, Fasting, Prayer, Earth, Mud, and others which are given for the well being of mankind.

CHAPTER XX (1-26)

Nevertheless, there remained many more sick people, that in spite of their fasting and prayer, still continued suffering horrible pain from their ailments. Filled with Faith, in the promises of their Life-Giver, they persevered in their fasting and prayer. There were some among the sick persons who, upon seeking to stand up to go over where the Healer was, got dizzy and fell to the ground. Filled with compassion, the Savior would approach them and console them saying that, if they would continue their fasting in prayer in complete Faith, they too would surely be healed.

However, one of them who was unable to get up, came out directly expressing his lack of Faith, saying, "Lord, is it fair that so many have been healed, and yet, we who have also fasted, prayed and been baptized (lustrated or initiated in Aramaic), remain sick?" Thus, the Anointed elucidated further, "Your ailments are more grievous than those who were healed already, because you have sinned a longer time than those healed: you have disobeyed the commandments of Mother Nature a longer time so you have to remain sick a longer time. But do not let that discourage you and keep persevering in your fasting and Faith, because, as things are, this is the only way you can get back your health. So that you may understand the necessity and importance of FASTING AND FAITH FOR YOUR HEALING, I am going to explain the way these kind and beneficial Messengers or Forces do the Will of Mother Nature.

When we fast, it makes necessary the need to not waste the forces and substances (in other words, modifies the functional economy of our organism) in our body so that it makes it possible to heal and cleanse our internal structure. Millions of little bodies (or cells, in modern language), of which your larger body is composed, have a work to do in changing the food you eat into the power of living, and when these cells do not get food, they get time to heal and repair the parts, or organs, of our body that are out of order. Other cells dedicate their time to the cleansing or hygiene of the blood, the flesh or tissue of the organs and whatever needs repairing. Now, these cleansing cells of the blood (or phagocytes in modern medical terms) seek to clean out the trash or garbage that accumulates within the human body, or Temple, by the natural gates and roads. But when the amount of rubbish is excessive (or today we say, the phagocytic index is high, in an analysis of blood morphology), they open up new roads of escape and gates on the surface of the skin, manifesting with oozing ulcers, skin sores, abscesses or tumors where the excess foreign substance can get out. In this way the skin sores, ulcers, abscesses, or tumors are not the ailments in themselves, but instead they are the necessary means of getting rid of the excesses, cleaning out or purging, in the healing or restoring health to the body's interior, provided by the All Knowing Internal Physician (Healer within one), which we have within our organism. Do not try to disturb, or interfere with the natural healing methods of this wonderful Physician who works miracles in healing.

Only when this Healer has finished his work of cleaning and healing what needed to be removed, leaving the body clean and healthy, does he proceed to close these escape gates in the skin, removing the ulcers, sores, abscesses and other skin ailments, which then heal, leaving the skin smooth and luxuriant. Such is the wonderful work of the Omniscient Internal Physician or Healer within, who is one of the Great Angels (or Messengers, Powers, etc. in Aramaic) of Mother Nature, who spontaneously carefully purifies and heals your body from within, without any need of any External Medicine-men or Physicians.

This whole, wonderful method of Healing or Salvation, (same Aramaic word is used for either) of your body was made possible due to observing this rigorous Fast. It is then when the Angel, or Power, of Fasting finishes his mission of healing successfully that some are permitted to return to eating again. Even then, the first days after a long fast one must eat light juicy food, allowing for a slow return to the normal more nourishing food one normally requires.

After this explanation of the importance that Fasting has in Healing your bodies, I shall now explain the very important part PRAYER HAS ON HEALNG or restoring Health. When you pray, you should be sending out luminous rays or emanations that are receptive to manifesting a renewed integration (or Wholeness) of your soul with God, the Great Cosmic Soul, that embraces or contains all that exists, and which is an All Moving or Omnipotent Center of Wisdom of the Living Power, of Vitality, Dynamism, Force, Goodness and Love. If this sincere Communion with God is sustained in all you do, accompanied with Righteous Living, good works helping others, kindness, and Love within an unbreakable FAITH, then your soul will identify with God, and He shall become One with you, and you shall become a channel of Blessings in Plenitude streaming from a Great Reservoir of Health, to provide Living Power to that weak and once-unclean body, charging it with vitality, energy and vigor, which shall rapidly restore it to health, both in body and soul. In this way you yourself shall be persuaded to also see the importance of Prayer accompanied by good works and righteous living.

Editorial Note: The Healer of Mankind forbade prayers of doubt, as the N.T. also shows, saying a prayer one should believe, anticipating reception of all one's needs thru one's commitment to worthiness and God's Providence,-the antiquated word "Prayer", associated with ritual repetition, being today better expressed by the mental act of Faith, or Affirmation of God's Omnipotent Omniscience. Thus, Prayer should be God Communion, acknowledging the Creative Law of Fulfillment, already giving thanks and praise to the Lord of Life, Health and Joy in Living for what we are so abundantly receiving. A beggar begs because he feels empty, unworthy, unwanted and consequently ever thankless, lacking in everything and abandoned to chaos and ruin by Orderly Cosmic Intelligence that is seen guiding every virtue of Creation and the Heavens. At first glimpse, it would seem advanced concepts about hygiene and healing could not possibly exist at the beginning of the Christian Era, but we have used both simplified and resourceful vocabulary of our times in alternate explanations of our translation, as well as realizing Hippocrates long before had also employed them. Too often, John, the Initiator (Baptist was used by Rome to hide his identity as the Gnostic founder of

Christianity) is looked upon as a simple credulous ritualist, when in reality he was the Sage who initiated his reform after a childhood life with the Essenes of Mt. Carmel with Colleges at Bethel, Jericho, etc. In that former incarnation, I experienced the same obstinate opposition that I have now in teaching the Vitalogical Sciences today, -with unknown tenets, and principles requiring such-will power in discipline opposing passions.

CHAPTER XXI

Let me remind you that, indeed, no one can enjoy Good Health, nor restore their health if they lose it, unless they comply with Nature's Laws. Yet, there are many who seek for health in vain by erroneous ways using drugs (in Aramaic remedies consisting of poison or venom are defined as drugs), scorning or despising the natural sources or the very fountain from which health flows in abundance. These children of error are blinded by the dazzling promises spread by the drug-mongers, who prey on the ignorance of the people, exploiting their credulity and diseases for their own gain, making it thus, the most profitable of all types of businesses, proclaiming that their cure-alls are miracle drugs that are infallible in curing diseases, which, altho being false, nevertheless is believed by the great multitudes of the population.

Hence, once more I must warn you that no one can heal the body with a medicine, because this would make void, or annul, all the wise laws of our Creator, which only grant health to those worthy of it, and never for the use of a drug. To obtain such worthiness or merit with God, one must comply with God's laws. Now, one of the listeners happened to be one of these drug mongers, or medicine men, who thus began questioning the Life-Giver or Savior, saying, "Master, you have said that other remedies never cure diseases. However, I have remedies that can make skin sores and ulcers go away, and that will take away headaches, toothaches, rheumatic pains and many others. Can you explain any difference between what I claim and the results I have, and those you claim and have in practice?"

The Life-Giving Healer replied, "Already I have told you, THE BODY HAS WITHIN IT A MOST WISE HEALING POWER, which makes for the Natural Defence and Powerful Resistance of the Human Organism. This Resistance consists of a great multitude of little bodies, or cells, whose mission is to maintain

Cleanliness or Hygiene and Health within our bodies. These cells, being living bodies, organisms, intelligent, complete, are capable of rapid mobility and agility, and yet they are too small to be seen ordinarily. We can all admire their wonderful labor when one gets cut, and we see the wound heal at once with such perfection that it appears the same as the healthy skin around it.

There are many kinds of cells: Of these, we shall only deal with the HEALING, HYGIENE AND MESSENGER CELLS. The Messenger Cells are the ones that advise us when an accident occurs within our bodies. This advice penetrates our consciousness thru pain which we feel in the region that is affected. For example, if a meal is bad for us, we have a stomach ache. Now, if you had the means of using your inner vision to see within your stomach right at that time, you would see Defence Cells in feverish activity. Also you would see Messenger cells carrying or relaying messages, one to another, by means of a network of informers, or nerves, which advise the central headquarters of leadership, or your brain, that danger exists. The brain, in turn, sends out its distress signal, or pain, that manifests that there is something regrettable developing therein. In this way you become aware of any trouble when it develops and you can help prevent this trouble by not eating some days. What I am saying, is that you naturally do not eat, or you fast, until the indigestion disappears. This means taking only pure water (living water, not dead tap, distilled or bottled water). Then you would see the Defence Cells are at the same time seeking to heal, to mend or to repair and make the affected part better, doing a perfect job. After it has been repaired, the pain will go away of itself, which is a signal that you may eat again.

Now, if the aforesaid inner vision remained with you, you would see the wonderful work of our Creator manifest in the Hygienic Cells at work cleaning out the body from within, carrying all the substances that do not belong there to the outside of the body, leaving them on the skin, which develops the kind of escape channel required, such as ulcers, eruptions, abscesses, pimples, and other ailments with skin symptoms.

In such critical times, there is a great need for PRIEST-PHYSICIANS or Healing Clergymen (We have no reason to believe Clergywomen were not equally in demand or more so.), who have the ability of counselling sick people because they have studied these Natural Healing Methods that we have briefly discussed, and who also comply with our LOVING ONE ANOTHER, out of the Charity in their hearts, would attend them mercifully and never for money. It is only on this condition that our Heavenly Father comes to heal our patients, and this factor was necessary for obtaining the successful wonders in healing that you have witnessed. If the patients were wisely instructed, so they would not fall victims of unscrupulous medical men who exploit the ignorance, the disease and the pain suffered by the people, such abuses making men rich quick could not come about. Due to this lack of a GOOD SAMARITAN HEALING CLERGY, Physician-Priesthood, or Medical Evangelists, (we add alternatives so as to not favor any), the sick are now forced to depend on these unscrupulous Black Magician Drug-Mongers, or Pharmacologists, who peddle their formulas, which for the moment, PUT OUR TRUE INNER HEALER TO SLEEP, or deaden the pain, so the signals of the symptoms of pain and disease disappear, including the eliminative skin irruptions. This is why such patients are contented with such wonder cures; believing they have really gotten healed of their diseases. Hence, we have the celebrated glory of these wonder cures and the Magicians who conjure remedies from such things.

Nevertheless, the new-found happiness is short-lived when the sickness that the patient suffers returns with worse evils. This is because the new-found medicine had only suppressed the EFFECTS of the Evil, so the evil could get worse. This is the RESULT OF INTERFERING WITH THE WONDERFUL NATURAL HEALING PROCESS OF THE INHERENT SAVIOR, the Healer within all or the Inner Physician (choice of translations again), worsening or aggravating the Cause of Disease. The SPONTANEOUS NATURAL SELF-HEALING OF THE ORGANISM was interrupted, and the medicines caused the acute disease to turn into a chronic and incurable disease.

You might be more convinced of this, if your inner vision could again penetrate within your stomach and closely observe the affected part. You would now be surprised, because in the very place where you had seen swarms of cells in diligent activity cleansing or healing the condition, you would now witness piles of little dead bodies, or dead cells destroyed or partially alive laboring under their heavy burden barely able to crawl. What had happened there? This was the Result of taking one of these ill-fated drugs, or this formula concocted by the trafficker of medicines, because all such remedies have, more or less in general, the basic quality of destroying the Natural Resistance or Immunity of the organism. The first effect of the destruction of this Natural Immunity, can be readily observed in the Messenger cells which stop transmitting warning signals, or causing pain, which is a grievous thing, because the patient does not experience pain and believes that he is well. So he continues to stuff himself with every kind of food, ruining his stomach, which causes bleeding ulcers, which eventually turn into cancers, resulting in death.

The Healing Cells, of this Innate Healer-Life-Giver were not able to avoid this disaster, because they, too, lie there wounded, and many of them completely destroyed. The same is true of the Hygienic Cells, for the same reason that they too lie incapacitated from performing their function cleansing within the body. Without the removal of these wastes, and the absence of the function of the Hygienic Cells that remove the burden of excess waste matter thru the escape gates in the skin, brings about the closing of these gates since they no longer have a function, and gives the appearance of healing the boils, ulcers, abscesses and skin sores with healthy, smooth and vigorous skin. These skin cells are far enough from the blood stream to receive the last of the effects of these deadly drug poisons, so that they still function to the last moment, altho with difficulty. The continued inner vision, if granted, would now be frightened by the horrible scene of the little dead bodies of dead cells rotting and decomposing in evil smelling putrification as the result of continued use of poisonous drugs.

Later, the bloodstream seeks to spread out these waste products, distributing them thru-out the organism, poisoning our most noble organs which start to fail in performance. The heart beat becomes irregular when one gets up too quick, one gets dizzy with black-outs, difficulty in breathing and what generally ends in heart failure, or partial or complete paralysis, and a premature death. This is the end result of the use of drugs, pain-killers and medicines in general, which at first relieve suffering, but later kill one."

Then, turning to the medicine monger, the Divine Master said, "This is my answer to the puzzling problem you gave for me to explain, so that you may be convinced that medicines, that you so highly acclaim publicly, do not heal, nor cure disease, but only poison the body. It does prove that medicines do not bring health, but instead give a worse disease, because their use converts the beneficial Self Healing Process into a painful evil, such as experienced in tuberculosis, chronic rheumatism, diabetes, cancer and even leprosy.

The truth of the matter is that the seemingly curing effects of some medicines are really so extraordinary that they dazzle and fascinate many learned men who do not know about the Natural Self Healing Process within our bodies. Those who know about the latter, know that the former is pure illusion, which accepts appearances for realities. Those who practice Natural Living know that due to VITALOGICAL LAWS, no medicine is capable of uprooting any disease. The only real natural resistance to disease, or immunity that is effective, is to keep the bloodstream immaculately pure, or Natural Hygiene. What a medicine really does is change, or transform one's acute diseases into chronic diseases, a beneficial evil into a corrupt evil, or a disease easy to heal into an incurable ailment. When it comes to creating a Natural Defence against diseases that invade the body, there is no medicine that can free, or immunize, the body from diseases caused by future plagues of infection. This is why no other True Method of Hygiene can exist, nor can it exist ever, because something that casts spells against God's Laws is not Natural, or Sorcery, whose Black Magic opposes the fundamental Laws of the VITALOGICAL SCIENCES. No drug can guard the body against disease or other evil, as Sorcery taught since old, but as again I repeat, it can change a beneficial evil into an unsupportable evil, because all that a drug does is deaden the body's responses, and suppressing the natural defence momentarily giving the impression that a person has been protected or immunized against diseases, when in reality, all that such sorcery does, is paralyze the Natural Hygiene or Resistance to toxins of disease.

Editor's Note: If it seems strange to readers that these principles, not only seem very modern or resemble Natural Hygiene teachings, let me remind them that that is because Hippocrates taught many of them hundred of years before John the Initiator, as did the Gnostic Healing Temples of Greece and Egypt. These Self Healing Hygienic processes are included in the Vitalogical Sciences; or Life-Giving or Saving sciences in contrast to Darwin's Biological or Life-Destroying or "survival of the fittest" chaotic theories of Biology. Instead of Sorcery, Magic, etc. that the Gnostic Christians of St. John, as well as the Essenes were accused of by the Church of Rome, the Roman Church did just that!

CHAPTER XXII (1-15)

There were many gathered there that marveled at what they had been taught, which for the first time they now had heard. Some of them pleaded to learn more about the new science, "Master, teach us more about the Internal Hygiene of Physiology of our body, so that we may know if everything within us is in order, that we may better care for our health and so we do not have to depend on these medical merchants that take advantage of our ignorance, and for each drachma in silver, poison us with their remedies which are worse than the disease. The Anointed One thus gave into their pleas, saying, Verily I say unto you, the number of the cells within your body are about as infinite as infinite as are the stars in the sky. Yet, all of them are absolutely indispensable for the correct function of our bodies. These cells are living beings, agile and dynamic, intelligent and rational. These little bodies are very much like the human beings they compose, because they are born, grow, reproduce, work, enjoy, suffer, love, hate, age and die to be replaced by younger cells.

However, among the human species, those who abstain from all vices, and observe the frugal VITALOGICAL WAY OF LIFE Close to Nature, there is the Strictest Discipline and a Perfection of Order even down to the cells composing their bodies, in this most wise regimen of the Best and the Most Capable. According to this Universal Law that binds the Ignorant, and gives Power to the Wise, also within the human body, Nature rules that these Microcosmic bodies (cells) shall synthesize the Universe, the Macrocosmos. Now within this Strictest Order, the Cells are thus grouped in Hierarchies (reflecting again the HEAVENLY HIERARCHY) each according to their Natural Capacity, specific tendency, affinity and mutual sympathy. The most vigorous cells, the most active and the most dynamic, the most intelligent, of themselves put themselves in the highest positions, with the most responsibility, and among the highest hierarchies. Accordingly, thus, the most intelligent cells form our Heart and Brain of our body, while the rest of the cells form the rest of the noble organs, the liver, the lungs, the spleen, the stomach, the intestines, the blood, the bones, skin, hair and others.

The cells of each organ are the best prepared for their particular work, trying their hardest to maintain their own organ in the best condition of function and most efficiency, but not solely for their own and exclusive profit, but always seeking to serve the best they possibly can the rest of the organs with which they are joined in close and inseparable interdependence. All these organs together form, in turn, a harmonious whole, or one great ORGAN, which is your body, just as the body, in turn, is a cell that forms the great Organism called Humanity.

This Cooperation, or Love of Order in Wisdom ceases in everybody when any individual, or group, disobeys the Laws of Mother Nature, giving themselves to the pleasures of city life, worldliness, vice and evil habits. Such is the life (first or second hand) of alcoholic drinks, the tobacco smoke as well as of other herbs (marijuana, etc.), opium and narcotic drugs, marriage-shattering prostitution or fornication, irregular meals eating all that the eye desires, followed by counter-measures in remedies and pain-killers, all of which make for sickness, weakness and degeneration of the cells of the participants, destroying their natural resistance to disease and dissipates all the vital energy. In such an organism, the Head of the Hierarchy in the Consciousness has been disregarded, losing supremacy over the disobedient cells, which thus begin to form centers of subversion called DISEASE, which causes the DEGENERATION OF THE ORGANISM, which can only lead to serious conditions such as tuberculosis, consumption, rickets, diabetes, cancer, chronic rheumatism, gangrene, leprosy, and so forth, which are the end result of cellular degeneration that ruins the whole organism.

This Lesson teaches us that one's well being depends on oneself. If we obey the Laws of Mother Nature we are assured of Perfect Health, material as well as spiritual prosperity, peace and Happiness. If one disobeys, one has to suffer the mentioned diseases, miseries and calamities without end. Also this lesson teaches us that we must follow the example of the cells of our body in our daily behavior, to identify in their Order and thus become the MOST PERFECT ORGANIZATION OF ALL CREATION. THIS PRISTINE ORDER OF PERFECTION OF CENOBITICAL LIVING, or cooperative common life among mankind, little by little, shall be adopted by all peoples as soon as they unite with the Hierarchy in the evolutionary plan of humanity. So, to be able to cooperate effectively in this strict social discipline, you should work with a complete dedication to Self Perfection, just as much physically, morally as Spiritually, but not only for your own personal and exclusive gain, rather always seeking to serve to the best of one's ability the whole of mankind, just as the cells of our heart serve all the body, and in case they rebelled and stopped working, the body would succumb totally. Just as there cannot be a deliberate paralysis in cellular activity within our bodies, so also there cannot be a paralysis in the social organization of mankind, and when we reach such a perfection,- this perfection being the supreme goal of mankind,- we shall reach our unavoidable destiny. This destiny requires that we keep climbing, on up to the snowy heights summit of Gods and Goddesses of the Heavenly Hierarchy, beyond earth, eternally. In this path, in the future, the most Enlightened and Cultured shall be considered those who out of Love and Free Will practice the greatest social justice, without resorting to the use of arms, strikes and blockades or a deliberate paralysis of work in progress, which in total constancy and good will cooperate with all including those most humble.

CHAPTER XXIII (1-10)

Then speaking exclusively to his own disciples, the Healer said, "Since you are endeavoring to learn the secrets of how to heal the sick, you must know how to manage this gift and guard this ability once you have attained it. It is very easy to lose it by abusing it, for example, when you EXPLOIT DISEASE AS A BUSINESS, as do the official medical authorities, getting immensely wealthy from the suffering of others and the misfortune or misery of mankind. To the contrary, you must not follow their methods. When you are in the presence of a person that is ill, ask the Highest to heal her or him. This is because of our own person alone you cannot make her or him to become well, since this can only be realized thru the Power of the Heavenly Father, who is the Maker of that organism, and thus, is the only One who knows how such organisms get out of order and how to heal them.

One should exemplify the GOOD SAMARITAN as a model, who had compassion on the man that robbers had left half dead, beaten on the road, healed his wounds, took him to an inn for further care till he became better, and then did not charge him anything for saving his life. To the contrary, he also paid the expenses for his rehabilitation out of his own funds. This is the MODEL PHYSICIAN (Healer, Savior, Hygienist, etc.) who should be the exemplar for Physicians always. However, if there are any among you, or those who come after you, who charge for the attention they give providing for the sick, whether this be in money, in donations or other benefits, they shall lose their gift of healing the sick, because God's Presence no longer remains in their actions. Every denarius (penny of N.T.) that anyone charges in exploiting disease as a business shall be converted into a thorn that shall forever pain such a person's conscience, taking away his joy of living. Under the True Divine Law within everyone's heart, such a physician is CRIMINAL, and as such, he is condemned to suffer the same misery, the same agony and the same pain in his next reincarnations, that he caused his patients to suffer, because the same unchangeable Law of Life, Healing also applies, stating that with the same measure that one gives, it shall be given back to one.

Editor's Note: In a May 29, 1951 letter, Prof. Edmond Bordeaux Szekely wrote that he had translated the most important part of "The Essene Gospel of John", which was only one-eighth portion of the full manuscript, which is obviously the one we are translating now, and that due to caring for 50 patients and other works, he could not take out a few months to finish translating the copies he made of the Gospel. He did give me the data needed for finding these Scriptures: "The number and file record of this manuscript is 156-P. I studied the Aramaic text in the Library of the Vatican, 'Biblioteca Apostolica Vaticana", under the care of Anselmo M. Albareda, Prefecto." Why was the complete version of St. John never translated or published? The answer became obvious when I finally found the Source thanks to the Samaritan Order, and read the above Chapter which accuse those who take money from sick patients as Criminal. Szekely had said originally that only two complete versions exist, one in Aramaic, and another in Ancient Slav. After 25 years passed since the above letter, he now gives a new story. So pressed for the remaining seven-eights of John's Gospel by students was Dr. Szekely that in Book II the name forgets John and becomes The Essene Gospel of Peace, with writings of Enoch, Moses, Dead Sea Scroll, etc., but no more of those harsh words of John concerning cure-mongers, and there is a Hebrew Source for the Aramaic manuscript. The Hebrew source is pictured with quotation, question and other punctuation marks which were not existent in those early centuries of our era, showing it to be the Professor's RECONSTRUCTION of what he selected as the most important part, only one-eighth of John's original.

As to the Discovery of the Essene Gospel, we read a new story saying he found them among the lost works of St. Jerome in the Benedictine Monastery of Monte Cassino, in Hebrew, and the Secret Archives of the Vatican, in Aramaic. No more about a common file-record number 156-P and Prefect Anselmo Albaredo; but now it is Monsignor Angelo Mercati as Prefect and his mysterious Secret Archives of the Vatican that Professor Szekely says he studied under in his new books. "Dust filled room with over 10 thousand packages of unexamined documents is a "terra incognita" that could never be proved not to contain the Essene Gospel of John, so why not search there for the answer. Why a new "Discovery" story by Szekely? Rancho La Puerta, from where Szekely wrote the letter to me, became "the largest health resort in America and the world", he owned the Golden Door (Escondido, Calif.), the most luxurious beauty resort in existence, an 80 acre meditation center (near San Diego) that someone called a "Spiritual country club", a dozen ranches in California and Baja California, a publishing business, several corporations, cosmetic laboratory, or a corporate empire that accumulated millions certainly speaks of success as a businessman. Never having met him, yet I lived a portion of his life thru friends working with him, at Natureland, Elsinore, Calif., rehabilitating the adobe stable that became Rancho La Puerta of this penniless idealist, as well as when those early helpers were refused visits because he was entertaining millionaires; his early printer inspired me to print my own works. Thus, virtually I had lived with him, racially being Hyperboreans (I of Finnish and he of Hungarian), we both lived joined in vows of Poverty, Chastity and Obedience in Catholic Orders (He a Piarist and I a Carmelite), we studied comparative eastern religions, anthropology, and in many other ways he contributed so that I was able to seek out the source of these mysteries, to tell you more of Christian origins. And it avoided the embarrassing need of him having to print this chapter of John's Complete Healing God Spell! In the end, possibly remembering the suffering of the sick one takes over to the next

79 The Healing God Spell of Saint John

reincarnations, he willed the corporate empire over to his wife and offspring, as an Essene contemplating Buddhist roots in his Illumination under an Oak tree, seeking to mend former religious vows.

CHAPTER XXIV (1-44)

Then, the Beloved Disciple, John, the Anointed of Spirit being the closest to the Lord, beheld and immediately prayed for the Lord's assistance, "Father, there is among this multitude, one so sick that he lies cast on the ground, faint with weakness, that even crawling on his hands and knees cannot come closer, but calls out, "Lord, heal me for I suffer greatly". For a long time the Healer sought within for an answer, having approached the helpless invalid, so that by inner vision he might see within the body of the patient for a diagnosis of the precise cause for his suffering. The body of the patient was emaciated so as to appear little more than a skeleton. The skin of the patient was yellow as a fallen leaf in autumn.

The patient contemplating the Presence of the Anointed, wanted to get up, but his weakness prevented it. With his eyes fixed on the kind Master he implored of him, "Lord, have mercy on me, heal me. I know you are the Messenger of God, and that you have the power to loosen my twisted members, and cast out Satan who causes me the torment within me. He gnaws at my intestines, he chokes me in my throat and he gags me when I try to breathe." One of the sick one's family added, "Master, I have seen this with my own eyes that he has the devil within his body, because I have seen this devil appear in the mouth of the patient while he was asleep. I saw his very face which was round, with big eyes and whiskers around his mouth. The Anointed nodded foreword, affirming that he knew what the man was describing. But John also then turned to the side where the group of his disciples who he was teaching the secrets of healing were, and explained to them: "It is not simply an evil spirit, or a Satan, that is lodged within this man's body, for this is an advanced case of hookworm. This worm got into this man's body years ago when it was less visible in form carried by unclean food eaten by the patient. Thru the years this worm lived lodged within the digestive tract, feeding upon the food that the patient ate. Thus after a number of years now it measures about 4 cubits. Now, after fasting a few days, the patient is greatly tormented by his worm, which from lack of food, hungers, and has become angry, tossing and coiling within his belly. With its fleshy gullet it bites and pinches the wall of the intestines and stomach, coming out as far as the mouth in search of food, sucking at the residues of old food still clinging to the intestines. When the corpulent worm finds no food within the body to eat, it may even appear at the mouth, or choke and smother the patient by stopping up the breathing passages. Since people are rarely accustomed to seeing such a thing, their explanation calls this worm Satan, so by this name I will have to call the hookworm so the multitude will understand me.

The Healing man, again speaking directly with the patient said "The fast you have been practicing for several days has given good results. By not eating for a few days yourself, also prevents Satan, your unwelcome visitor, from eating also. This is why this guest has become so tormented, causing your body to become the Cave of Satan, rather than a holy Temple where God may dwell, all because you once ate some unclean food making you the host or carrier of this visitor. But do not fear, because Satan shall be destroyed before your body is destroyed. While you fast and pray, the Angels of God protect your body, and Satan shall be overpowered by the Divine Power of these Angels." This greatly impressed those present with such revelations of the Divine Master, and they besought him, saying, "Master have compassion on this helpless invalid, for he suffers more than all of us. If Satan is not cast out from his body soon, we fear he will not live to see tomorrow."

The Christ answered, "Great is your faith. By your faith shall your prayer be answered. Soon you shall see Satan, face to face, his frightening countenance, and then you shall all be convinced as to the power of the Angels of God when they cast Satan out of the patient.

Immediately, Jesus milked a mare, a she-ass, that was grazing nearby, and the milk in the earthenware pan heated by the sun gave off the aroma of fresh milk when placed under the nose of the patient, and the Anointed then said: "Behold, the three Angels of the Lord shall now perform a miracle which you shall witness with your own eyes. The Angel of Water rules over the essential component of milk, and the Angel of Sunshine shall warm it and the vapor of the milk rising up shall enter the patient's nose, being draw within by the lungs, and consequently the vapor shall enter the devil's own nostrils, which will please Satan because he esteems fresh milk especially. And so it happened, because then the milk's vapor in the pan heated by the blazing hot sun began to rise, it filled the air with an agreeable odor.

The Christ held the head of the invalid in his lap, and brought the earthenware tray closer to the patient's nose, saying, "Breathe in deeply so the Angels of Water, Sunshine and Air within the milk's vapor re-possess your body, and cast out Satan. "The invalid breathed deeply of the milk's vapor rising from the pan of milk. Again, the Anointed encouraged his patient further, saying, "Now, do not lose faith, there is no need to despair, because Satan shall immediately leave your body by your mouth, since he is overcome by hunger because you forced him to fast several days. Summoned by the welcome odor of fresh milk, he shall come out of hiding to partake of the warm milk, because FRESH MILK IS THE FAVORITE FOOD OF SATAN.

Then suddenly, the body of the patient was seized with ague as he sought to vomit but could not. He gasped for air but could not breathe, causing him to faint, as the Healer held his head and held open his mouth to the air. Now pointing to the mouth of the invalid, the Healer-Savior in John said, "Look within the patient's mouth, because you shall see Satan already coming out". They all looked as he bid them, and to their horror, and astonishment, they all saw Satan slowly, and cautiously, coming out of the fainted victim's mouth going straight into the pan of milk. Then, the Savior took advantage of this situation and beheaded the aforesaid Satan, which was pulled out of the patient's helpless body which the abominable beast had tormented for so many years, the victim recovered his breath, breathed deeply and cried with tears of joy. With great difficulty, he even got up on his feet and walked a few paces. He was filled with happiness to see he really could walk again. His strength returned, his cloudy vision turned clear, and thus he was able to see clearly his Savior, the Anointed of Spirit, who with a loving smile looked upon him.

So happy was the Savior for having been able to help this helpless victim, that he rejoiced with him, observing, "Look at this great beast that has been lodged in your intestines, how corpulent and well nourished, it was, because it fed from the richest part of the food you ate, leaving your body thin, under-nourished and without strength to work. Now that this may not occur again, you must not feed upon such abominable foods as you did before, so that your body may become pure and clean. Then, it shall become a Temple of the Lord, your God, who shall live within you in the dwelling of your heart.

All that were gathered there were filled with Joy and marveled at the Wisdom of the Anointed, and they said, "Master, you certainly must be the Messenger (Angel of the Holy Spirit) of the Lord, for you know all the Secrets to removing illness and saving health. The Newly Saved One, over all the rest proclaimed praise for the Wisdom of the Savior, and came to cast himself down to kiss his feet as they all cried tears of happiness.
Editor's Notes: It is an outstanding characteristic of the Healer in that so far he has not used medicinal herbs, or other medicines, to heal the body, but instead he has used the Angels, Powers or forces of Nature such as Water, Sunshine, earth, air, fasting, prayer, etc. The Kingdom "Edessa", the first Christian Kingdom, was ruled by the Gnostic Christian Church, because, King Abgar, was brought up with, and shared the beliefs of Bardesanes, Gnostic theosophist of the Valentin school and great student of Hindu doctrine, reincarnation, Karma, etc., also he defended the Christian Faith so manfully before representatives of the Roman Emperor (then still "pagan"), that Epiphanius called him "almost a confessor." Bardesanes taught, "From Nature cometh growth and perfection of the body. Nature ordains that old men would be judges for the young and the wise for the foolish." King Abgar wrote the Healer, "Jesus Christ, who appeared in Jerusalem:" "I have been informed concerning you and your healing performed without the use of medicines and herbs" beside offering him an invitation, "my city is indeed small but neat and large enough for us both." This chapter is also a foremost example of why Gnostic sects received Serpent titles, such as Nassenes, Nass-Aryans (Nazarens), Ophites, etc., which the Church of Rome accused of Serpent Worship. In this case, the hookworm is the Serpent, Satan, which Jesus casts out of the Temple (our body), as well as a deeper understanding of the N.T. Bible story of Jesus casting out the Money-changers and flesh-mongering Physician-Priest Corporation, that Jewish Rulers pretended to be, just as today the State accepts doctrines of flesh eating, drugs, usury as legalized robbery by our bankers, etc. taught as the State-Religion. Also interesting is the data that condemns FRESH MILK as "the favorite food of Satan". Even many babies have an allergy

against using fresh milk, which is no substitute for breast-fed nourishment from their own mother's milk, as do adults. Yet, milk is included as one of the foods, along with fruit and herbs, that God gave for man's food in another chapter (Chapter 33), showing that ripened milk, like ripened fruit, is to be used, in the form of clabber or bacterially cultured milk. The tiny bacterial plants cultured in milk, restores the intestinal flora and augments disease-resistance (phagocytic index) enabling toxin neutralizing beside producing enzymes.

CHAPTER XXV (1-19)

Then, the Anointing God-Spell left them, instructing John, "In your care I now leave this flock. I shall return on the seventh day of fasting and prayer, to join in with those rejoicing because they persevered to the seventh day. After these seven days of fasting and praying, the Heavenly Blessings reaped were very rewarding for their perseverance. All the pain and agonizing complaints had disappeared from those who had been ailing miraculously and instead they were proclaiming the wonders of healing they had experienced.

On the last day, the fasting and prayer came with a happy and rejoiceful commemoration. The magnificence of the dawn contributed greatly to the solemnity of the gathering. Not a cloud darkened the heavens. The sun rose with great splendor and brilliance. When this King Star had fully appeared on the horizon, with astonishment all of them witnessed how the figure of the Exalted and Anointed (the Scripture could be mistranslated as "Christ Crucified" from Aramaic alternatives) descended still circumscribed with brilliant illumination, even more dazzling than the sun seemingly, floating down to them from the mountain top. (This figure of circle and cross gives the esoteric symbolism of this God-Spell allegory in the New Testament hidden in the crucifixion myth). Finally, when the magnificence of the Anointing Spirit came close with outstretched arms, the Radiant One greeted them. No one dared to say a word. In awe, they could only cast themselves down before him and kiss the hem of his garment (a hemless garment) as a sign of admiration, honor and thanks that they deeply felt for healing their ailments.

"Do not thank me", he told them, "but the Highest One who sent me. He made all that is and has being, including Mother

Nature (symbolized in the origin of Adam and Eve in the Genesis story) and her Angels that serve us, if with obedience and repentance, in fasting and prayer, we ask for her intercession (service, meaning of Virgin's intercession in the Catholic rite). And suddenly it seemed the Anointing Spirit was bidding them farewell, asking them to return to their homes. Blessing them, he said, "Go in Peace, and sin no more against Mother Nature, because this is the only way to be healthy without pain and disease."

However many responded, "Master, where shall we go, when it is so good to be here? We do not want to leave you, because you alone radiate Peace and Happiness, that which elevates our Spirit and gives us Joy in Living. Master, tell us, what are the greatest sins against Mother Nature, and what shall we do to avoid them and maintain health." The Anointing God-Spell (Ecstatic One leading the Assembly, Ecclesia, as St. John was doing) responded, "Your Faith in me certainly is encouraging. So I will tarry with you a bit longer, and he began to tell them about the Virtues, what people should practice, and the sins they must avoid to live in Happiness without disease and pain for a long life.

Editor's Notes: We cannot just read these Scriptures once to understand them: All that is being said takes years of repeated study and meditation, comparing them to the N.T. Bible, the Church liturgy, Eastern Scripture and life's many aspects of experience (material, mental, spiritual, etc.). Each one of us has a great deal of this stored in our Cellular Genetic Memory or Heart's Intuition, but Perfection requires the whole process. Each person has blocks or blinds that stop them short of understanding fully, wanting to be as well as being the Pristine Perfection of Paradisian order, a Heavenly Oneness in All.

All these Scriptures and tales, including N.T. allegories were masterpieces of Gnostic Wisdom, celebrating the Heavenly Triumph of their Master and Savior in Consciousness, in which they see him ascend and resurrect into exalted glory of the True Light of the World. To the Initiates of their Gnosis, they did not pretend that Jesus Christ was a man ever, for as the N.T. reads: "Where there are 2 or 3 gathered together in my Name, there am I in midst of them." That fact is most evident in this Chapter of the Healing God Spell, in which the Anointing Spirit is seen leaving and again gloriously returning to rest upon him, after the wary trials of taking care of fasting patients for 7 days. The Spiritual Light Body manifests condensed in Life's experience as well as extending to Heavenly Exaltation, yet more often than not, it is invisible to the uninitiated (prejudiced, etc.), and not that God ever leaves an Initiator like John. One no longer speaks of their individual body, but all credit goes to His Name, The Anointed Savior (Jesus Christ) within one, when one acts or thus speaks teaching the God-Spell, altho not visible in the many chores of daily life.

To know how the original God Entrancement, or Book of Illumination (gospel) really started, let us observe that the oldest Peshitta N.T. did not contain any genealogies for Jesus. A Hebrew writing, as claimed for Matthew's gospel, should start with a blessing, but it has none, and a genealogy would be at the end, never at the beginning, showing that this was a fraudulent insertion by Papal Editors of the Roman Church. The Spirit of God, Christ or Savior needs no Jewish or Roman genealogy. Jesus was the son of the Beloved or "David".

When did the separation of the Spirit of Jesus Christ, resting upon and associated with John, the Initiator (also called "Baptist" or Founder in varied Aramaic translations) of Christians, and a separate so-called "historical man" named Jesus Christ of Nazareth (or Nazarene) occur? Certainly at the Council of Nicea (325 A.D.) there was no disagreement, since there "The Holy Catholic and Apostolic Church Anathemizes those who say there was a time when the Son of God was not," it resolved. It was clear enough, the Son of God, Jesus Christ, is Eternal, not a Jesus that is born or dies in time. The Disciples of John, Founder of Christians, did not claim exclusive rights to that Eternal Spirit, altho they knew his Gnosis manifested it, and he said it came about after his experience of the dove resting upon him while baptizing on the Jordan. The Christian Church had no "Apostolic Creed" until it appeared in a common prayer book in 600 A.D. None of the early Fathers up to the year 400 ever mention it, but a careful study shows to the contrary, even creeds opposing reasoning as to an intangible Spirit, incapable of proof, except myths of tradition and allegory, which eventually gained popular belief among opposing parts, resolved by accepting compromises to have peace in an embryonic Holy Roman Empire.

It was not until Jerome (Je-Rome, God-of-Rome) produced the Latin Vulgate version of the Bible, after 400 A.D., do we learn of a man named Jesus, with two different genealogies, of 28 and 42 generations, claiming the Holy Spirit to be his Father, along with a long line of Jews and pagans as well. The Latin Vulgate did not become the official version of the Church until 1546. Before this fictitious version, the Gospels started by telling of John, the Founder (Baptizer) of Christians, who after his 29th birthday became known as the Healer, henceforth called Savior (Jesus) Anointed (Christ) of the Holy Spirit. Now, the Church of Rome didn't care too much what Christians believed, since they only sought to be authoritarian Compromisers, to keep Peace in the Empire and prevent religious uprising against Rome. Each one of the Gnostic Schools had sought to become the official doctrine during the first few centuries, causing a spirit of discord that Rome felt made her Empire insecure. Origin openly affirmed that Josephus who had mentioned John the Baptist, did not acknowledge Christ, in that Christ and Christian were later adopted as titles at Antioch. Justin Martyr, Clement of Alexandria, etc. affirm the same fact.

Then in the 5th Century, Nestor, the Patriarch of Constantinople, brought the "historic" human named "Jesus Christ" into being. Not being philosophically or mystically inclined, he opposed the doctrine of "Mary, the Mother of God" for he believed that Jesus was like any other man, but a little more virtuous than most men, and not the co-equal of the Almighty and Eternal. George Lamsa, who presented me with his autographed Peshitta New Testament in 1953, held that the Church of the East was the Nestorian sect, but is his English translation of the Peshitta, "pure and simple" as he defines it to be? He also adds the Latin Vulgate style genealogy of Jesus as a son of Joseph, showing later college training (Canterbury, Oxford, etc.) misled him into such folly. Nestorians are of the Chaldean Church, not being the Eastern Church exclusive.

This made for the division of the Eastern Church, the Monophysites being the opponents of the Nestorians: The Monophysite Patriarchate of Antioch roots from the First Christians, which founded the "Christian Church of Syria, Iraq and India, the Patriarchate of Alexandria with jurisdiction of Christians in Egypt and Ethiopia. In modern times we have charge of the Patriarchate in Ecuador. "Jacobites" are the best known Monophysites, named for Jacob Baradesus. Like Dioscoro and Cirilo, he believed Christ was God, but was not a perfect man. If a perfect man were God, the nature of God is man, but God and man are not of the same nature. Monophysites means those holding God has one nature, substance or attribute, which is Eternal, Incorruptible, the Light or the Word, and thus cannot manifest as a mortal being, born, dying, suffering, as claimed of Jesus Christ as historical man or individual. Yet, in many occasions, even for extended periods, Jesus Christ has dwelt in the human frame as a temple, or vehicle, but not that all men dwell in God, or God dwells in them manifestedly, because Christ signifies the Anointed of the Holy Spirit, while Savior means one who saves or heals. St. Paul and St. John both teach this doctrine in the N.T. Bible. But Nestor appealed to the materialist who needed to justify human virtues, and thus he advocated teaching that Jesus was a good virtuous man, a model for others to follow, not just a Spirit or state of Illumination, thus developing the belief that Jesus was a mortal man, separate from John, the Initiator of Christ and Christians. Thousands of books have been written on this question, but they are arbitrary concepts, or the result of the Roman Church forcing compromises in dogma on the world, first in Ecumenical Councils and then in its Canon of Scriptures inspired by God or the Holy Bible. One cannot legislate and compromise God, Truth, or Spirit. This is why the direct followers of John, the Initiator, known as Gnostic Christians, Nassaryans (Nazarenes, Nassenes, etc.) have a "John Book" that states: "After the death of John, the world shall fall a prey to error. The Roman "Christ" shall overthrow the peoples, the twelve seducers shall travel the world. He shall corrupt John's sayings, pervert his Initiation (Baptism) of the Jordan, distort the words of Truth, and preach fraud and malice thru out the world." The Salvation of mankind depends on restoring this Truth, it says.

All of the above indications makes me wonder about Prof. Szekely's affirmation stating in the 1937 Preface to the "Essene Gospel of John": "Nestorian priests, who under pressure of the advancing hordes of Genghis Khan were forced to flee from the East towards the West, bearing ancient Scriptures and ikons with them", as to the origin of his two versions, that is, the Aramaic Version in the library of the Vatican and the old Slavonic version at the Hapsburg library. It seems strange that the Nestorians,- who believe Jesus was only a good man, and not God in nature,- would carry with them Scriptures that tell of the blinding intense

Light of the Anointing Spirit floating down and ascending up to the Heavens. That only one-eighth of John's original was permitted in the versions Prof. Szekely obtained, shows that the 7/8ths or missing portion has not been published in English and other Szekely books because the contents were censored by the Vatican Papal Authorities that he studied under possibly.

Instead of 4 Gospels in the N.T. Bible, there was only one, the 4 coming from the same original, to which interpretations of translations added details enhancing the stories. The earliest record of Christian Scriptures found in the Library of Congress, Washington, D.C. was made by Charles Waite, affixed to the Gnostic Gospel of Marcion (Marc-John) dated at 128 A.D., and contains only one Complete Gospel with ten letters or Epistles of St. Paul, nothing more, the rest being later additions. Irenaeus decided that there should be four Gospels like the 4 winds. Marc-John translated the original Aramaic Version into Greek, the Latin Version being made by Luke or "Paul's physician" or Corrector (one giving remedies) later known as Censors, Matthew's Gospel making it conform to Hebrew prophecies, and John's Gospel, Epistles and Apocalypse are a part of an original Gnostic Gospel completing Marc-John of the Sayings or Teachings. Another aspect of the study reveals that all four Gospels are portions of the same Gospel or Teachings that are now separated into 4, which the Initiate must Restore.

In discovering the Keys to God's Kingdom, we soon find that the original God-Spell, or Initiation of the Illumined was for Gnostic Christian followers of Saint John, the Initiator, and that the full teaching is revealed in the parts of a MANUAL FOR INITIATES now scattered in the New Testament, other Gospels and Epistles collected by the Gnostics. The Christ, Jesus are both titles, referred to also to with "Lord", "Master", etc. as already explained. Rarely does John refer to himself, because all the credit belongs to God, Spirit, Truth, Light, the Word, or the Name of God manifest, Savior, Anointed of Spirit, and not the mortal flesh person, mentality or ego, which are ever-changing and ever evolving. Christ, Buddha, etc. are not persons essentially, but rather refer to a State of Consciousness in Cosmic relationship or Divinity. Nor can we pretend to Name or Describe God with Words, only indicating paths to Truth. Thus, John called himself a Disciple of Spirit, Light, Word, etc., the Son of the Father in Heaven, but worldly Church teachings have presented John as merely a humble Messenger, heralding another person named "Jesus", while possibly John saw "Jesus" whenever he gathered together with one or more disciples, for "there am I in the midst of them". "Baptist" in English now only refers to a washing, sprinkling or bathing ritual, but it originally meant in Aramaic one who Initiates disciples, or is the fountain-source of Illumined Teachings. As the Gnostic "John Book" says, the Roman Christ defrauded mankind.

Altho Jerome admits he used a Latin Version made before him, he did not reveal its true contents defending Roman doctrines. This was the VETUS ITALICA or Old Latin Version which scholars prove precede Jerome nearly 200 years, having been made about 150 A.D. from Aramaic originals. In 1066 an Old English translation of that Vetus Italica was outlawed by the Papal Church authorities because it had "all the Hebrew and Chaldee (Aramaic) words translated", this being made from a text Gregory, the Great, sent to England by St. Augustine in the 6th century and used for teaching by the Early Celtic (British) Church. Because such frank presentation of revealing truths would do away with Papal subjection to Rome, Latin was made the official language of Papal Church teachings and English versions outlawed. There were 99 words called "Sacred" because it revealed the mysteries hidden in the N.T. we now have, but became "an eyesore for the Popish party". The papists doctored even English words, such as changing God Spelle to "God Spelle" with accent on the "o", so as to read "Good Spelle, Glad Tidings or News. God Spell was just that, God Entrancement because it was the Book of Illumination Initiation. This is not strange because Buddhist Missionaries, called "Essenes" (the Pure, Healers) or "Gnostics" (who know Wisdom) were spreading the teaching of the Great White Brotherhood in Palestine, Syria and Egypt, in compassion seeking to free their peoples.

Another of those 99 "sacred words" is "Baptism", which could have been revealed to mean the Sunrise or Illumination of the Initiation that John, the Initiator (Baptist) taught. The Teacher of Illumination, the Enlightened, was John, and thus, the Papal authorities hid it by translating the Aramaic as merely meaning the "Baptist" or bathing-ritualist! John, the Enlightened was prophesied by Siddhartha Gautama Buddha to come 500 years after him, so he was John, the Buddha, as well as the Anointed or

Illumined of Spirit, or Christ. The Essenes and Gnostic Christians greeted the sun at Sunrise with their arms outstretched, gesture of prayer, which made the outline of their bodies resemble a cross encircled by the illumining sun, the symbol of the cross circumscribed by a circle the code of their life seeking Buddhahood or Enlightenment, as well as the Living Tree of Life and round fruit being the source of the Living Water that gives birth to PARADISIANS and the fruits of Spirit, Truth and Fulfilling God's Plan.

In fact, "John" is sufficient in itself, without "Baptist" explanation of meaning: Yohanan in Aramaic being composed of first suffix "Yo" (like Hebrew Je) being the abbreviated form of the Sacred Name of God, meaning the Ever-Existing One, or "He-Who-Is" (That which is), the very meaning of "Tathagatha" or Buddhahood, as well as "Hu-kikat" of Sufi teaching. In the Christian Bible, often the "Lord" is substituted for God, the Highest Name being Unspeakable or too holy for the profane to utter. The second part of John, Yo-hanan means to invoke or be "Endowed by the Spirit of God", Anointed of Spirit (Christ) or God's Grace, all of which again must be defined as the Illumined, or the Buddha in Eastern terms of Sanskrit and "Ju-Lai" in Chinese. By reading "New Light in an Old Lantern" by Joseph Bonner we learn many of the these esoteric secrets now hidden in archaic Bible versions of our day. The New Testament means God's Covenant Anew of Ancient Teaching Restored, being the Book on Illumination or the God Spell of Saint John, or Illumined Buddha as well as Christ, Savior. The Translators and Copyists censored by Papal authorities made all the versions of Aramaic Scripture conform to their dogma, rather than seek the true meaning. Even the Greek words took on so many meanings to conform to Church doctrine, "but" having 12 meanings, "by" representing 11 English words, "for" 24, "in" 15, "of" 13, "on" 9, "master" 6, "Lord" 16, and so on. "Christ" should read Anointed meaning Endowed of God's Spirit, "Son of David" should read "Son of the Beloved", "Thomas" altho translated "Twin" but means Spiritual Double, Matthew (Mathetes) refers to Disciple. The Old English, and Old Latin versions never used "Jesus" which now is interpreted as a name of a man, but stated meaning to be "the Healing man", "the Healer", giving our title "The Healing God Spell of St. John", in Eastern terminology being the Healing Illumination of a Holy Buddha.

It is not necessary to stop with "John the Baptist", or study any special Holy Scripture, or join any of several opposing religious bodies that I have united under my leadership (Gnostic, Catholic, Orthodox, Buddhist, Yoga etc.) or any tangible, physical, historic entity or movement. All of them are only vehicles designing paths to Spirituality, to be described as a Consciousness, Spiritual Principles, Truth or Order of Cosmic Scope, beyond all materialistic sensual or intellectual evaluations. Even John could be done away with by critical analysis, either as an insect (locust) eating loafer, who robs wild bees of their honey, dressed in a camel-skin, who rebelled to honestly working for a living as a demented wildman stirring up political rebellion, or as we have almost reached to show John could really be an Aramaic equivalent for the Buddha, Illumined Christ, whose message the missionaries from India sought to instill among the people of Palestine to prevent further bloodshed as opponents of both the Roman political rule and the Jewish religious hierarchy. What we are really working at in our modeling, sculpturing or mentally exemplifying is not some physical, tangible, mortal human or body of followers to be torn apart by clever critical minds, but rather the realization of a new Spiritual Consciousness. To realize this Spiritual Consciousness, Cosmic Thankfulness, Living Joy of Loving all, Inner Sunshine even on cloudy days so that one can stand firm and not be tempted by each passion to abase or demean those we love or do not love, and not fall into errors damaging our own lives and the lives of others by our actions, or lack of action, spiritually oriented scriptures (such as our Healing God Spell and the critical and analytical explanation of widely accepted Scripture often stirs up alternate avenues of being, and even living like a new-born Divinity!

CHAPTER XXVI (1-20)
THE HEALING GOD SPELL OF SAINT JOHN

Our Heavenly Father created the earth, the heavens, stars, suns, -planets, and all that exists. When the earth was ready to receive human life, God created the first couple and placed them in a delightful PARADISE, called Eden, here on earth, where these children might nourish themselves from the luxuriant trees producing delicious fruits. This Prehistoric Paradise was situated in the land of flowing waters (Nile is indicated as one). Divine Messengers were put in charge of this first couple. Eventually, in the midst of Eden they built a statue for lasting reminiscence of their destiny, which had the body of a Lion and the head of a woman. This was to symbolize the Ascension of the soul from the lower kingdom to a higher kingdom, from the animal kingdom to the human kingdom. This is the humanizing of the brute, bestial animal part within mankind. In time this first couple began to multiply greatly, from which the races of mankind were derived. The color of these first inhabitants was golden, or white slightly toasted by the sunshine.

However, this color was modified when some of earth's inhabitants were located in cold regions of ice and snow, since the color of snow became the best defence against the cold environs. In turn, those who went to live in the torrid regions of the burning hot sun, little by little became darkened, taking on a black color which is the best defence against burning heat. This is because both heat and cold can cause injury, which brought about a cold pigment, white, like snow, and a torrid pigment, black, like charcoal. The Heavenly Father loves all his children, regardless of what color they may be, and he sent them Masters of Wisdom, Guides, Messengers and Prophets to teach them.

The First Great Commandment the Heavenly Father gave mankind was to LOVE THY GOD, Thy Lord, with all your strength, with all your heart, and all our soul. The Second Great Commandment his children received was to LOVE ONE ANOTHER as you love yourselves. When he indicated one another, this was meant to include every living being in Nature, because they are included in God's Creation, all of which should be respected and protected by mankind. Love even your worst enemies, because only LOVE can extinguish HATE in whosoever you hate, turning it into Love. But if you continue hating one another, this only increases hate in the heart of others so as to never eliminate it, and seriously damages both.

We should Love all Mankind, all people, because they are Brothers and Sisters, Children of God, and of the first parents, Adam and Eve, because even if the color of their skin is different, whether black, white, copper, red or yellow, he loves all his children. In emphasis I repeat you must love your enemies, considering them as your best friends. Bless those who calumniate you, do good to those who injure you, love those who hate you, give food to those who throw stones at you, pray for those who hate, damage and persecute you, because all this really means you love God, and one another as you love yourselves.

CHAPTER XXVII (1-18)

Love Thy Father and Thy Mother, because this also is a very important Commandment. This will give a long life of health and happiness.

THOU SHALT NOT KILL, is another Great Commandment that the Lord gave mankind. Since all Life was given by God, no human has the authority to destroy that which only the Highest can give. He who destroys the Life of someone else, even if he is a king, a judge or an enemy, is an evil doer, a CRIMINAL, in the face of Immanent Justice within our being, which sooner or later will balance our deficiencies, as tho it were written in indelible letters in our Living Book of Life, or our eternal genetic record. He who destroys the Life of another in reality destroys his very own life, in that it prepares the same kind of death in his own life. Whosoever kills or destroys animals by eating their flesh, causes this flesh to turn into a poison within their own body, poisoning oneself and producing disease, a life filled with habitual failings, afflictions, menstruation and pregnancies and a painful death. The pain and agony, the fear and terror that man produces in animals when they are slaughtered, sooner or later, will produce the same agony within those who partake of their flesh, according to the LAW OF JUSTICE AND LOVE (Law of KARMA), described within the axiom, "With the same measure that you have meted out to others, you shall be measured."

Flesh is a detestable food, a poison with the power of poisoning the bloodstream to its last drop, sooner or later causing painful diseases, and a miserable early death. When the animal is slaughtered, it suffers mortal fear, shivers, groans, overcome by terror, that produces a cold sweat, the sweat of death, which is a powerful cadaverous toxin that becomes the root cause of the deadliest ailments, that lurk, laying in wait for mankind, because it upsets all the physiological functions within man's body. Of equally deadly consequence it alters every psychological faculty, eventually even bringing on the complete loss of one's mind. On top of all this, it alters the functions of the heart, stomach, the digestive organs, the vision, hearing, smell, taste and one's higher sensitivity. For instance, if your nose loses its normal sense of smell and savor, so that one feels a great repugnance for certain salad vegetables, it is a sign that one's nose does not smell things right, in putrid perversions, because Nature does not produce foods that smell bad, but instead they should always be of pleasant aroma, attractive to the appetite. The normal healthy sense of smell in full and perfect function enjoys the aromas of vegetable salads.

However, to the contrary with the lower vibrations of animal flesh, along with their emotions and passionate feelings of their bestial nature which can transform a man who eats their flesh, to re-live or assimilate their psychological nature, lowering such a person to the passionate feelings, emotions and the desires of these animals. Such humans become worse than animals at times in their behavior in blood-thirsty ferociousness and aggressiveness, so they no longer have any conscientious scruples as to killing, and even provoke bloody participation in slaughter and massacres. The majority of all military conflicts are provoked by men who act like animals, worse than ferocious beasts. Then one of the disciples, knowing it troubled many, brought up the question, "Master, if it is forbidden to eat animal flesh as a food, what should we eat?"

The Christ responded: "OUR HEAVENLY FATHER HAS SAID, "BEHOLD I HAVE GIVEN YOU EVERY KIND OF GRASS THAT GROWS IN THE FIELDS, EVERY HERB, ALL GREEN PLANTS AND VEGETABLES THAT GROW IN THE FARMS, GARDENS, AND EVERY KIND OF FRUIT THAT GROWS IN YOUR ORCHARDS OR GROVES FROM WHICH TO SELECT YOUR FOOD, BESIDE THE MILK OF YOUR ANIMALS, FOR THE USE OF ITS CULTURED PRODUCT. Eat not flesh and blood that lives in animals; it is Sacred, to be respected, for to do so trespasses against the Supreme Law that "THOU SHALT NOT KILL!"

Editorial Notes: The reader will observe in the paragraph just quoted that the Samaritan Scrolls rescued from the Alexandrian Library,- in contrast to Prof. Szekely's Vatican Version,- do not contain the confusing censored interpolations, in which the purpose of seeds in propagating plants (of Genesis 1:12) is confused with the purpose of green plants and vegetables, beside that of fruit and trees, being for the food of mankind (of Genesis

1:29) along with the bacterial plant product of milk alone. In other versions Bible Scribes were able to hide the identity of the Forbidden Food of the Garden of Eden, in that seeds were intended to propagate plants alone and not to be used for food, which brought about man's destruction of forests to grow grains and other seed crops that eroded the soil creating the Gobi, Sahara, Arabian and other deserts, beside reduce man's longevity after taking to a diet of bread from very near a thousand years to only 120 years. With this cunning confusion everyone is able to justify bread-eating: God gave us "every herb bearing <u>seed</u>" for food, but with the Samaritan Scrolls there no longer remains this cover-up recourse to self-delusion. Later, the Samaritan Codice will show how seeds or grains are to be used only to make vegetables (or fruit trees), and not to be used for food in their concentrated form, just as integral whole milk is to be used soured for its cultured product, clabber, but not to be used as fresh milk, which is for calves and the "favorite food of Satan". Since seeds reproductive substances, intended to reproduce "its kind" as Genesis states, when they were eaten by man and woman, they caused shame, woman having a fetid running ulcer shedding blood each month, and man becoming a belligerent victim of passion causing excessive population problems and violence as a way of life, to give expression to his sadistic bestial instincts craving sex and cruelty for pleasure. Alexander, Hitler, Mussolini, Bolivar, etc. not only were great warriors but also vegetarians. God accepted Abel's offerings of dairy products, but condemned Cain in conscience for building a desert by eroding grain-growing, beside becoming the First Murderer in Sacred History, as the consequences of grain growing and bread-eating. When milk is used fresh it is adapted for calves' nutritional needs, not those of man, and thus transmits animal psychic attributes while endocrinal components remain intact, which must be broken down naturally by ripening, or allowing bacterial plants to transform the animal product into plant protein which, like fruit and vegetable juices becomes directly assimilable by the body. Thus, clabber is able to immediately regenerate the intestinal flora, saving the life of those in whom it was destroyed by the use of drugs, pesticides and food intoxication.

 As to the Original Paradise, Herodotus, the Greek Father of History, held that the Hyperboreans in northern East Turkistan (Altai-Baikal) were the first dwellers of "the Cradle of Mankind", as we describe in "VITALOGICAL ANTHROPOLOGY". Quoting from the "Egyptian Book of the Dead" we illustrated how the Egyptians, and Atlanteans before them on Thera and Krete, also held their origins to come from a "golden race" of Tschudic (Finnic) Aryan origin in a gigantic white race with turquoise blue eyes like the Heavens just as the Aryan "Zenda Avesta", and the Taoist Chinese Scriptures all concur, along with the Pre-Inca tradition who speak of the Vierachochas as their origin being like white foam on the blue seas. The Pristine Order or GREAT WHITE BROTHERHOOD of Central East Asia, as well as the WHITE FRIARS of Mt. Carmel Essene Colleges, are all described as the Spiritual Guides and Architects of mankind's Heavenly Origins.

The Gnostic First Christians of Antioch from the Johanine and Alexandrian tradition, (as described in my Patriarch Archbishop Apostolic diploma), along with the Essene Order of Mt. Carmel I also can speak of from Apostolic tradition, just as I do for the Great White Brotherhood, Lodge and Order of Gurus of Tibet, and they all point to a Buddhist origin, beside N.T.: the Three Wise Kings or Magi of the East (Matt. 2:1). Yet Philo of Alexandria describes the doctrines and origins of Essenes and Therapeuts as being of northeast India named "Gymnosophites" as Buddhist-Yogi missionaries due to "naked Philosopher" attributes. Describing our "PARADISIAN" principles in "The Order of Paradise" (Copyright 1962), we gave direct Apostolic Origin to the Essene Order of Mt. Carmel, which relies upon Philo's "De Vita Contemplativa", as one can also see in our "INNER ORDINANCE OF THE HEAVENLY HEIRARCHY", as well as St. John and Genesis.

In these Rules of Contemplative Life of what Philo calls "Wisdom Lovers", the meaning of the word Philosophers, the copy in Mead's "Fragments of a Faith Forgotten" we read: "Indeed in Trismegistic (Hermetic) literature we find a number of distinctive doctrines of Gnostic Christianity, but without the historic Christ, and all these doctrines are seen to have existed for thousands of years previously in direct Egyptian tradition, especially the doctrine of Logos, the Savior and the Virgin Mother, second birth and final union with God." Therapeut colonies had crowds in every Egyptian Province, beside Greece and Palestine, which gives a Greek origin to our word Therapeutics, Therapy, etc., but not only did they pretend to heal the body, but their way of life was designed to heal the soul, just as Jesus means Healer and the word Essenes means Healers of both body and soul. All the traditions of the Ancient Catholic Church of the West, as well as the Eastern Orthodox, agree as described by (1) Eusebius (Father of Ecclesiastical History), (2) Epiphanius and other Earliest authorities, (3) Cardinal St. John Newman (most famous English Theologian) and (4) Johann Dollinger (most famous German Theologian) and others, in opposition to Papal Infallibility proclaimed in 1870, being for "De Vita Contemplativa" which teaches a frugal life of discipline, growing your own vegetarian diet for sustenance, allegorical view of N.T., Christian exegesis and Theology, beside the fact that Eastern Christianity outnumbered the West during the first millennium. Thus in our search for origins, rather than Jerome who assembled the Latin Vulgate Bible which Prof. Szekely relied on for doctrines to give a Vatican Church of Rome perspective, we have included Johanine, Samaritan and Alexandrian panoramic views.

Moses was an Egyptian with a name of royal origin, as Sigmund Freud points out in "Moses and Monotheism", who was initiated in the deep Egyptian Mystery School which means that the "Book of the Dead" gave origin to the Ten Commandments, and the contemporary Pharaoh ascended the throne in 1375 B.C., just before the Exodus. Moses derived his doctrine of Monotheism from Amenhotep know as Ikhaton of the 18th Dynasty of Egypt who preached One God, One Faith infallibility to keep a vast Empire extending to Syria-Palestine politically united, as Roman Christianity imitated. It started as Aton, and Adonai meaning "Lord" or "Father" of Jesus as the name for God, altho the Jews adopted Jahve (Yahve or Jehova) from the God of volcanic displays of Sinai and Arabia, giving the terrible and lower character they desired to express their vengeance. Thus, armed with a mean God of war, they lived in gory war till they had conquered a vast "Promised Land", sacrificing animals as their only rite and for food in psychopathetic worship.

CHAPTER XXVIII (1-7)

After these final words, everyone remained silent, save one who formulated a new problem: "Master, what if a ferocious wild beast attacked my brother in the forest, and was about to claw and kill him: Should I let my brother perish or should I kill that ferocious beast? In this case would I not violate God's Commandment, "Thou shalt not kill", if I killed the ferocious animal?

The Anointed answered, "Since the beginning of the world it has been said that among all the creatures that inhabit the earth, man alone was created in the Image of God. For this, the beasts shall be subject to man, and not man subject to beasts. Therefore man is not transgressing the Law when he has to kill a wild beast to save his brother. But he who kills an animal without cause, just for the morbid sport of killing, or for its flesh, or fur, or skin (leather one should not use), or for its tusks, such a person indeed has violated God's Law of "Thou shalt not kill". It certainly is a truth that whosoever slaughters innocent victims, sooner or later shall receive just punishment, because the soul of the slaughtered animal shall lie in wait to seek revenge, and in any coming struggle shall favor (or karmically compel) any assassin's sword, or similar circumstances, to destroy the life of such a guilty individual just as he killed the original victim.

CHAPTER XXIX (1-21)

"Master, Moses, the leader of Israel allowed our forefathers to eat flesh of clean animals, and he designated the beasts that are unclean which were forbidden for food", remarked one listener who still held a doubt concerning flesh being a forbidden food. "Master, would you remove this doubt within me concerning flesh eating. You prohibit the eating of all flesh of animals, yet Moses allowed some to be eaten. Which Law comes from God, yours or that of Moses?"

Jesus then replied, "Our Heavenly Father gave us the Ten Commandments thru the teachings of Moses for your forefathers to honor. These were severe laws, wise and unchangeable for a people of a more advanced or higher evolutionary maturity. But the people of Israel were not ready to understand or obey these Commandments. So Moses prayed to the Lord, saying, "My heart is heavy with sorrow for my people are like little babes with infantile minds, and are not able to understand your Ten Commandments in their literal meaning, and much less in their Spirit. So allow me, oh Lord, to modify these Ten Commandments with new interpretations that are within the mental capacity of being understood, and then broken down to something that has a capacity of being taught, practiced and obeyed. Then, when they have progressed to a higher level of evolution of greater understanding and maturity, they shall understand and obey these original Ten Commandments of your Law in all its integrity, both in the literal meaning and in their spirit. So Moses broke the stone tablets whereon the Ten Commandments were written, and for every law therein, gave ten explanations to make them more acceptable and easier to follow in the daily lives of dull infantile minds. This gave them ten times ten commandments.

When people stray farther and farther from God's ways, the more and more laws they need to govern them, which also means the more and more steps or grades they need to reach God. The reverse is true also, in that the closer people get to God, the less laws are needed. In other words, the less steps they need to reach the Highest, until no laws are required, no steps remaining in the stairway because one has fully ascended into Divinity, one with God."

CHAPTER XXX (1-27)

They all listened to grasp each word and then remained astonished by the wisdom of the Savior's explanations, but when he finished, they begged him to go on, "Tell us more, for we are anxious to learn about all of life's mysteries which you alone are now revealing to us.

The Savior consequently went on teaching them: "As I have just illustrated, these-ten-times-ten commandments thus have been arbitrarily compromised so there existed exceptions to "Thou shalt not kill" in the rigor sense of the Word. Altho this commandment prohibited the killing of every sentient being, in the mentioned case we discussed, and in other emergencies, men have arbitrarily allowed for the killing of animals, but not humans, because these people were so low and gross in the scale of evolution." This answer at once brought up the question: "Master, if there was this reason for killing animals, then what were the other cases or reasons for killing animals, when killing is allowed?"

The Spiritually Anointed responded: "Certainly there seems to be a Cosmic Reason which I shall try to explain. Life is also ruled by Ages, Cycles or Periods. A Cycle is like the time or period of infancy in the life of a child, when he or she lives happily in the parental home where he/she need not work, find food, clothing, shelter, toys and affection. After the child has grown out of the period of infancy, it enters the following period, the period of adolescence. Thus, it has become time for the child to prepare and leave its happy parental home to go work outside, earning his food by the sweat of his brow.

The same thing happened in regard to the Life Cycle of Mankind, which in its infancy resembled a child in its infancy. The first inhabitants of earth lived happily in their Paradise on Earth created by their Heavenly Father, without any need to work because all their needs were taken care of, without a need to struggle to get food for their table. But when they had grown up or out of this Paradisian Infancy, they entered Adolescence, having to abandon their Eden, to go populate and cultivate the earth which the Creator had prepared for their need in evolution, to make them earn their daily food by the sweat of their brow. They remembered so vividly their Divine Origin, which had been so sweet and delightful, when they were able to know and converse with their Heavenly Father, just as carnal children speak with their parents, and this memory (genetic intuition) remained so impressed in their minds that they did not forget it since. The truth of genetic intuition in all envisions this happy, innocent Paradisian State when one needed not to work, having one's Holy Table provided for by the Lord whenever one needed food. With these wonderful memories remaining unforgettable, ever enduring in their minds, in tears they begged that their Heavenly Father would let them return at once to Paradise where they had lived their happy infancy. Of course, this made it hard for them to concentrate on their earthy work, or at least face the hard battle for self survival, to earn their own subsistence, cultivating the land.

So this their Heavenly Father did in his Omniscient Wisdom, making it possible for them to forget their disturbing memories by submerging mankind in a deep slumber, that made them unaware of their Divine Origin and glorious past. To do this it was necessary to bury the Divine Spirit in a solidified dense earthy substance of human embodiment thru the eating of foods that make this possible. Now, the best foods for this process of making the human body more dense and gross are all flesh foods and alcoholic drinks. These foods allowed the Divine Spirit to dwell in a human embodiment so dense that it could not manifest its Super-Conscious State, but instead, only its lower materialistic manifestation. Such mind-dulling, stupefying drugs or narcotics, of which animal flesh and wine are only examples, (since they include L.S.D., marijuana, tobacco, medical drugs, agro-chemicals in foods, etc.) so cloud the human spirit in density that not one ray of spiritual sunshine can get thru to revivify the spirit buried therein. All this came about as the Eternal Selfless Divinity within mankind transformed little by little into the transitory human personality, of a lowly gross existence of selfish earthy being. Consequently human beings lost their insight as to the purpose of life on earth, and the glimpse or intuitive knowledge of what awaits mankind beyond in the magnificent heavenly realm or planes of being beyond physical existence.

Losing contact with his spiritual insight with knowledge of the Higher Self, or Enlightenment, man's mind became earth-bound, sub-human, with all the faulty characteristics of a lower being, with its hate, selfishness, resentment, wars, haughtiness, vanity, vices and evil habits of a bestial personality when it remains buried and engrossed in matter. With this greater density of embodiment hiding the Spirit in gross matter, the Highest was able to accomplish the need of letting mankind forget its Divine Origin, his home-sickness and brooding tears about losing his Paradise on earth. Thus, in time he even denied that such a Paradise even existed, speaking of it only as a fabulous legend. The people of earth were engrossed in earthy works, cultivating land, breeding cattle, fishing and other tasks, that they had no time to talk of days gone by, or the possibility of any higher state of life on earth." Just as soon as the Healer explained these things, one of the Disciples inquired, "Master, is there any hope for a better future for mankind?"

CHAPTER XXXI (1-22)

The Messiah and Healer replied, "The Heavenly Father has sent me with this wonderful message of the Heavenly Realms, or Kingdom of Heaven, that shall soon be restored to earth. If you want any part in this Kingdom you must make clean your robes, garments of the soul, so they shall be immaculately spotless and white like fallen snow and flowering lilies. In other words, what is needed is a Higher Way of Life, and Honoring the original Commandments of the Lord. Now is the time for good works, showing you really repent your past errors. Only those who overcome shall be allowed in the Coming Heavenly Kingdom.

The human race has already gone thru the lowest eras or ages in the Cycle of Evolution, descending the deepest it could go into materialism, and henceforth started scaling to a happy return to the Heights of a Heavenly Paradise living in the Spirit of the Heavenly Father. For this Ascension, the human organism needs to be unburdened, freed from its useless ballast or overweight. The ballast was needed to enable mankind's descent, but now for the Ascension it becomes necessary to get rid of or lighten the load on ship. This requires the dematerialization and rarification of the human body substance, which is a process just opposite of what was needed before to materialize and to make it dense. Since that came about by the eating of animal flesh and drinking alcoholic beverages, now in the upward cycle of mankind this becomes a burden since it prevents further ascension, making it necessary to get rid of the excess ballast. Thru this densification and rarification of the human embodiment, mankind has become conscious of what is needed and his part in living in the New Age of Mankind's Life Cycle in the Spiritual Age already at hand.

Let me emphasize, now is the time to let loose and take off, or free the Spirit of all this heavy matter in the gross physical embodiment of mankind, making it lighter or subtle (Sattwic is the Yogi name for it), since this is the only way to lift up our True Being and soar up to the Spiritual Heights, and return to the Paternal Home from which mankind has strayed to acquire the deep knowledge and experience which Life has given humanity.

To eliminate this heavy gross embodiment under which our Spirit is smothered, means First: to not eat any more slaughtered flesh, nor any other slaughtered animal product. More directly, you must not participate in the slaughter of any living sentient being by eating of the products of its carcass. As I have been teaching you, YOUR FOOD SHOULD BE FRUITS AND VEGETABLES. Along with this requirement is also the tenet that you should not drink alcoholic beverages. The juice of grapes taken right after pressing without fermentation is an excellent beverage which gives strength (if taken alone in the place of food) and does not produce drunkenness, as happens if it is used after fermentation which produces intoxicating alcohol. The best of all beverages and the purest Living Water is provided in Nature, in the mentioned foods, which cannot be improved upon or substituted for by non-living or inorganic beverage substances used by man. By this process of purification working thru both the physical organism and the Spirit, mankind shall awaken from its millenniums of slumber, which the Heavenly Father has brought about to make man's progress possible. By practicing this Spiritualizing Dietetics, Vitarianism, exclusively, you shall start to have a glimpse or foresight beyond this present world into the wondrous world or realm which the Heavenly Father has prepared for those who are worthy of a life of greater glory, enriched by past earthy experiences, knowledge and wisdom in your return to your Heavenly Origin."

Then, speaking especially to the disciple who asked for a clearer explanation as to why the Spiritually-Anointed-One prohibited the eating of animal flesh, which Moses had allowed, and which one of the Laws, whether those of Jesus, or those of Moses, came from God, the Savior said: "From the detailed explanation I have just given, you should be able to understand that both Laws came from Gods, those of Moses and mine, their differences existing only due to two distinct Periods or Ages of Mankind, for which they were designed. The earlier Law of Moses prepared for Man's decent into materialism, and my Law for the New Age in the Spiritualizing or Ascension of Mankind."

CHAPTER XXXII (1-40)

All of the listeners remained Spellbound by the Wisdom contained in this explanation. Taking advantage of this, John besought within himself to continue, breaking the silence by formulating a relevant inquiry, and then letting the Anointed Savior speak the answer thru him.

"You will be asking the Lord within yourselves, as you contemplate these Teachings of Wisdom, who is the true authentic Messenger of God but he who is known both by the Supreme Wisdom he teaches, as well as by what he eats and drinks. If he eats animal flesh, and drinks alcoholic beverages, and calls himself a Messenger of God, accordingly such a teacher is a Hypocrite, a deceiver and a liar, which must be the case with Simon the Magician. Is that what our Lord teaches?"

Then the Anointing Savior or Healer ("Jesus Christ") answered thru John, "Such an interpretation is MY TRUE TEACHING. (The meaning of the word ORTHODOX). The Sacred Scriptures confirm this to be True. When Daniel and his companions became God's Messengers before King Nebuchadnezzar, they intuitively could not accept the stimulating mouth-watering spicy flesh meats prepared for their delight, nor did they partake of the intoxicating beverages of the King's table, but instead they only partook of the most frugal foods, FRUITS AND VEGETABLES, which, when eaten uncooked, contain within themselves the purest living water for thirst.

They strictly remained true to this Divine Intuition without defiling their bodies, which maintained them pure enough to have the sensitivity and strength to not lose their Higher or SUPER-CONSCIOUSNESS, and thus remained capable of receiving the Spiritual Guidance they then needed. In this way they retained their Spiritual Gifts and the contact with the Highest, which made them the Great Sages of their time, and the Divine Messengers and Prophets who even amazed the men of Wisdom of their day. These Divine Teachers keep their physical and Spiritual Bodies Immaculate, pure, clean and sensitive, so as to receive the clear and full Guidance of the Most High, and thus arranged that the right things would happen at their auspicious right time. The Divine Faculty of SPONTANEITY which they enjoyed was not only due to their strict, pure, vegetarian diet, but also because they lived strictly on LIVING PLANTS, VITARIANISM, just as Mother Nature teaches us, without destroying their LIFE-GIVING PROPERTIES. Just as I also have taught in my Commandments for you, so also Daniel and his companions became DIVINE APOSTLES (word for Messenger and Apostle used is one in Aramaic) because they strictly obeyed the Commandments of the Most High (Living God of Daniel, Shadrack, Meshach and Abednego.) Only if one practices the highest human virtues, that is, if one lives a frugal life based on pure, holy and righteous living, sincerely dedicated to hard work, in an unselfish way promoting the material and moral well-being of mankind, shall you receive the highest honors or Laurels of the Living Crown, and be SPIRITUALLY ANOINTED as an Apostle and Faithful to the Most High. (In Aramaic this word for Anointed Spiritually Celebrated, made merry or rejoiced, as is the meaning of Christ, Messiah.) Since this path of Supreme Sacrifice is long, troublesome and wearisome to really reach the Supreme goal, everywhere you find false prophets, teachers who falsely pretend to be the Faithful of the Most High, and even seek to demon-strate their claims by practicing the evil art of BLACK MAGIC. (Opposite of true Magi, or Wise).

For this, they evoke the spirits of those who have died, with whose aid they are able to produce raps on doors, cries, move tables and chairs or other objects, so as to attract those who are not cautious and are easily impressed making them believe that they really possess occult powers. However, only the lowest spirits, those of infantile souls, and quite often in many cases of the subhuman spirits, lend themselves to such manifestations, but never the truly respectable and advanced spirits. It is because these ethereal spirits are composed of very subtle vibrations (like aromas, etc.) so they are incapable of any kind of manifestation in this gross material world.

To make them manifest, these Black Magicians make use of the physical bodies of those who assist them in sessions, secretly drawing out an immense reserve of one's VITAL LIFE FLUID or Force, without their victims realizing what was being done. However, this Vital Force is what gives Strength and Energy to man. With recourse to this energy, the invisible spirits are able to conger up these Spirit phenomena.

Just like a tree wilts, withers, dries up and dies if its vital sap is tapped and totally drained, so also a human being will soon pass away if one continues to lose their vital force. This is why it is very important not to assist in such waste of the Vital Forces, or, in other words, it is dangerous to participate in spiritist seances. Those who assist exhaust their Vitality until they are weak as if they had done the heaviest physical labor, or climbed a steep mountain. If they continue to assist in such dangerous seances, they can lose all their reserve of Vitality, becoming obsessed, demented, paralyzed idiots or crazy.

However, this is not the worst that can happen to the unwary friends of Spiritism. These mischievous spirits may take over the homes of the dead mediums, haunting their houses till they are uninhabitable. The most precious objects become theirs to enjoy and play with, only to take pleasure in smashing them and doing the most damage possible. There are cases where these spirits also possess the domestic pets, such as dogs, cats and goats, so these animals become able to walk on their two legs, either backward or forward, just like human beings, causing mischief for humans. They may even obsess your bodies, without you being able to prevent it, so that you start doing all kinds of dishonest and repugnant things against your will.

Nevertheless, there is a way to cast them out. These spirits are also very timid like a small child. They may be frightened away with the use of spiritual weapons, choosing those which are sharp, piercing and painful like knives, spears, and especially swords and sabers. All you have to do is make believe you are engaged in sword play with them, swinging your saber over your head as if you are attacking your imaginary invisible enemy, crying out, "Get out, you evil spirits!", so they are obliged to leave the premises in terror. However, if these spirits are persistently established in a place, you have to resort to more effective means. In such cases you have to resort to the most potent means of exorcising all these evil spirits and get the best results. That Most Potent Power is God. All the inhabitants of this home invaded by evil spirits, should go on a fast for a few days, continuing to pray with the Faith or vision that the Heavenly Father will come to the rescue, and if they put this in practice, Almighty God will surely cast them out. God has put impassable gates between this world and the world beyond, and these gates should never be forced open by unworthy, immature humans. These gates can only be opened by those worthy of possessing the KEYS TO THE KINGDOM OF HEAVEN. All of you can get these Keys someday, and you can get them fasting and praying, doing good works and behaving in the way I teach you." (See Matt. 16:19-22, 17:20)

Then the Divinely Anointed began showing how all of this relates to the UNFIRED LIVING FOODS DIET. "Since Living Foods contain the most sublime essences found in Nature which are derived from the combination of sunshine, air and water (beside soil), their composition is so delicate and fragile that they are easily destroyed or can evaporate, simply by cooking them. Thus cooking these Living Foods deprives human of their sublimest essences which contain indispensable mental and spiritual energies and substances, which make possible man's development on the higher planes. Cooked food only feeds the physical body, while Living Food not only nourishes the physical body more completely, but also the Spiritual Body, the brain, and the mind wherein dwells the Intelligence, Wisdom and the Higher Concepts necessary for advanced attainment. Editorial notes: Not only does one squander away Vital Force (gained by living food, Living Breath, etc.) in Spiritist Seances, but those who masturbate and waste away sexual fluids continuing to have reproductive losses and orgasm, likewise invoke the subhuman spirits, which drag one lower and lower, and thus are not even able to ever get on Living Foods, and well up their force to become Spiritual Joy to become a Fount springing up into Life Everlasting. Also one will note that certain people use others spiritually to gain their own ends, which leaves them exhausted, so that their presence, conversation, etc. in cases can reduce a victim to a skeleton by such vampirism. They are weak willed in their own hearts, and thus use up one's will power undeservingly.

While it is true that the New Testament Bible did develop into one of Mankind's Great Masterpieces of allegorical narrative fable, and does give morally impressive instruction, yet it has historically been used to foment wars, political persecution, and the very opposite, offensive characteristics by righteous fanatical dogmatists. Just like the saying of wise men in proverbs and politics, gossip and selfish manipulations forever on the lips of the worldly multitudes, the Bible became a mixture of all those to satisfy Rome's desire to control its Holy Empire by universal creed.

In our "INTRODUCTION" (pages 3-6), beside Editorial Notes (p. 25, 26, etc.), we illustrated how SIMON MAGUS, not only made himself the scape-goat of Roman Religion as the founder of Gnosticism, hoping the critics of Catholicism would adopt his doctrines, but they use the kernel of his teaching as the Gospel Truth for the Chair of St. Peter or the Pope. Due to my own revelation after Heavenly Baptism or Initiation giving Birth to the New Age as Father of the New Race in 1942, and after reading the New Testament being convinced that Christ's death was a hoax or of deeper significance allegorically, believing that my mission was Resurrection of John the Initiator, I can see just how Simon pieced together the first Gospel of Jesus. Simon was a disciple of John Baptist, but John's teaching had opponents saying he did not fill the public tradition and Jewish scriptural prophecies on the Savior. Young Simon, in envy of his teacher's popularity, and subconscious desire to be the answer to the expectations of the public, suddenly became convinced he was the Savior answering the problem. John, as we shall later explain, received the Gnosis of his teaching from the original Sanskrit "Golden Text of the Holy Grail" (to give it a label), which

Buddhist Yoga Missionaries were spreading in Syria-Palestine and Egypt as "Essenes". Simon kept this as the mysterious Gnosis heart of his Gospel, and then filled in the prophecy tradition by Eastern Reincarnation theory that he had been the Zealot Josephus mentions seeking to uproot the Scribes and Pharisees with a virtuous life but also using the sword, for which he was Crucified. This creates a split personality ideal, Simon ready to cut the soldier's ear off as the N.T. narrates, and John's enviable virtues of not killing anything, so we have the Anointed Savior Resurrect in John, and Simon Peter, his Rock of Faith but counter-virtue of bravery ready to give his life for truth and justice in the flesh. The subconscious rapidly invents the scenery and characters for dreams, giving birth to visions and the ingenious scheme of the N.T. The mystery of "I bring thee not peace but the sword" and all kinds of allegories all begin to be pieced together, in rivalling Apostles, John and Simon Peter of the N.T. but fulfilling the Old Testament in Gnosis or Holy Spirit Incarnate Universally. The Church of Rome cites Simon for saying he was the Highest Power (God Almighty), who appeared in Judea as the Son (Jesus Christ) in the story of the Crucifixion, then in Samaria as the Father and other nations as Holy Spirit. The Church of Rome had only to invent the legend that Simon was only trying to make himself into another Jesus, but the Gnostic Initiates know that Simon was the author. But the Allegories of inner debate, flesh and spirit within us all, were like the Arjuna-Krishna debate the battlefield of the Bhagavad Gita, so why spoil the Mystique of the Gnosis with expositions?

CHAPTER XXXIII

The Healer pursued even profounder perspectives by explaining, "The Commandment 'Thou Shalt Not Kill', must be understood as including also 'THOU SHALT NOT KILL ANY OF THE FOOD THAT NOURISHES YOUR BODY',- not only giving you muscular strength, but also mental power, so that your mind is clear, alert, able to grasp concepts and assimilate them, enabling you to understand and put them in practice. One needs to eat Living Food because ONLY LIVING FOOD GIVES LIFE, since it quickens both body and soul, and acquires sensitivity of Spirit, or in brief, gives you physical and intellectual power. Living foods take away the boring stagnation of mind, bad temper, evil characteristics, pessimism, and moreover become sunshine that brightens one from within, so that which has darkened can be illumined. They replace gloom with gladness, obstinacy with affection and happiness, grudging and hate with friendliness, sincerity and willingness to help others, pessimism with optimism.

LIVING FOOD GIVES LIFE AND THE JOY OF LIVING!

In turn, Dead Foods bring Darkness within you, extinguish one's Spiritual Vision, so everything becomes obscure, gloomy, making one a pessimist, bored with life, aggressive, seeking to hurt others, hostile, not allowing anyone to live in peace and finally making oneself very ill, suffering aches and pains, so as to die prematurely. A very WISE LAW OF MOTHER NATURE STATES: FROM LIFE COMES ONLY LIFE, AND FROM DEATH COMES ONLY DEATH! Everything that deadens and kills your body, darkens your insight and destroys the Spirit within one.

Do not eat what has been killed by fire, frost or freezing, because fired, baked, boiled, frozen and rotten foods also shall burn your body, freeze your blood circulation and scald your body, just like a plant that is watered with boiling hot water. Be not like the foolish farmer who planted cooked wheat: His fields bore no grain losing his entire crop. Be like the sensible farmer who planted living seeds, which brought forth vigorous plants and a good crop, yielding a hundredfold increase.

Eat only Living Food such as the FRUITS of your orchards, the plants or vegetables from your gardens, and the ripened (clabbered) milk of your animals, without cooking them, because the same Infallible Wisdom of the Lord which made your body, also made Living Foods appropriate for nourishing that body. All the fruits are the most healthful when they are fully ripened. The Creator knows best how to prepare food (without cooking) using only the warmth of the sun, which does not cook vegetables growing in the garden, fruit ripening on the trees, or the milk ripening in a crock, only vitalizing them, seasoning and coloring them with solar energy, which becomes the Vital Force that moves our bodies, giving us strength and health. The elephants, the camels, horses, oxen and others that are the mightiest beasts that tread the earth, generally graze only on green grass. What better confirmation is needed for the TRUTH IN LIVING FOODS BEING THE SOURCE OF ALL LIFE!

CHAPTER XXXIV

Immediately, some who were gathered there, nevertheless persisted in asking: "Master, how can we prepare our daily bread, without wheat nor fire?" They knew John lived in the desert, using no other clothing but that which grew on trees and ate no other foods but that which grew of its own accord in the wilds (carob husks, berries, buds and tender shoots of plants and trees), but they could not believe such a life was for them and their families. No meat, no bread, no wine,-what indeed remained in life for them to look forward to?

The Oracle of Healing responded, "The sun is the greatest source of heat, of power, health and Life. Without the sun, the whole earth would turn to perpetual ice and snow. The sun provides all the heat that is ever needed to prepare your food. Listen and I shall tell you how to make "Living Bread". (Bread and meat mean food in Aramaic: nourishment)

First soak a portion of the seeds from any select seeds you have (wheat can be used for quick results if other vegetable seed is inconvenient), in an earthenware tray so the angel of Water may enter and moisten the seed. If the tray is placed in the sun, then both the Angel of sunshine and the Angel of the Air shall penetrate the moistened seed and awaken, revivify and start newborn growth in the seeds. To realize the natural (genetic) purpose of the seed selected and of all seeds, plant the seed and keep it well watered after planting, so it can grow the green vegetables or grass or plants you wish to eat. These vegetables and green grass are a delightful and agreeable health food in this form used as a tender salad vegetable, giving them their greatest nutritional potency, and fulfilling the natural (genetic) purpose of growing green plants for food. (See Genesis 1:12,29)

These vegetables, wheat grass or selected plants may be liquefied if they are crushed with appropriate stones, pressed in a wooden press or squeezed thru a cloth, much like one pressed juice from grapes and fruits.

To eat crushed grains in wafers would be like your forefathers in coming from Egypt, and bringing with them their slavery to flesh pots and bread-eating habits. Even if you put the wafers in the sun from sunrise till it reaches midday to turn them over to remain until the sun sets to be fully scorched by the heat, as they did, and leave them there till the morning dew gives them their sweetness like honeycomb to please your palate, making them tender to chew, all this was and is of a clouded understanding, since it produces not only a lack, but the destruction of living solar energy by the prolonged hot withering, scalding and baking of the plant food in the sun all day, killing the food. It is without any doubt that the Angels of Heaven which make seeds, sprout and grow green vegetables from them, also know how to prepare our daily food without baking any dead bread.

Celebrating the change of the seasons, in times of need or other emergencies, you may have to use sun ripened and dried grapes, fruits, vegetables dried green in the shade, or honey to have something to share with your friends or guests.

The Heavenly Father and Mother Nature provided Fruits and Vegetables for our Holy Table (Missa, Mass, etc.) as our daily food and drink, and which we shall graciously receive in thanksgiving (Eucharist) if we understand and Love our God in heart, mind and soul. This food is the true Heavenly Manna because it is the Living Bread cast down from Heaven and therefore, as Living Food, Fruits and Vegetables contain the delicate and subtle essences (vitamins, enzymes and minerals) which make them whole, complete and true Living Food. Being prepared by the Heavenly Angels, with the natural intensity of solar fire on plants growing with roots in the moist earth they live to become part of the strength, vigor, health and long life of our bodies. Only such growing and living food can be wholesome because it contains all the nutritional ingredients and essences the complete living body requires.

This was the kind of food that yielded 969 years of life to Methuselah. This same living food maintained the pure and holy (Essenes) who freely made the Exodus from Egypt without the long 40 year war conquering the wilderness. It is the source of the Immense Power developed in the workers who ate thereof to be able to transport and lift those enormous blocks of stone into place building the pyramids ages ago in Egypt.

Publisher's Note: Here is the English translation of the Spanish version using a word for word translation, which differs from the translation done by Dr. Johnny Lovewisdom.

Chapter 33 of the Spanish Version:

1. Various health-seekers asked at the same time: Master, how shall we cook our daily bread?

2. Jesus responded: The sun is the principal source of heat, energy, health and life. Without the sun the earth would be a ball

of ice or snow. This same sun gives us the precise temperature to cook our bread.

3. Listen attentively and I will tell you the procedure to cook your bread with the sun.

4. Soak a portion of grain, that could be wheat, barley, rye, etc. in a porcelain pan so that the Angel of Water can penetrate inside the grain and make it soft.

5. Place the pan of soaking grains immediately in the sun so the Angels of Sun and air infuse the grain with their beneficial forces, enlivening and awakening their germinating force that sleeps within all seeds.

6. Keep the grain moist and in the sun until it sprouts. These green sprouts have an agreeable sweetness like honey and because they are vegetable sprouts they give the grain a higher nutritive power than regular unsprouted grain.

7. Right away while fresh, grind the sprouted grain in a stone or metal mill until it is converted into dough.

8. From this dough make thin cakes like our parents did when they fled their captivity in the plateau of Pamir.

9. Put these loaves or cakes in the early morning sun and keep them there until the sun reaches its highest point at midday, then turn them over so the other side can be embraced by the Angel of Sunshine, and leave them there until the next morning so that the calm of the night and the morning dew completes the job giving the cakes an agreeable flavor like pancakes with honey and a smooth softness on the palate when you chew them, the softness is produced by the dewdrops.

10. If it is cloudy with little sunshine, you can extend the cooking time another 24 hours.

Note: Where there is little sun (nowadays in the modern era of Aquarius) you can use electric or gas ovens to imitate the same temperature as the sun in order not to destroy the germinative power of the grain that makes up this bread. To find the right temperature take some of the spouted grain that has been put in the oven and then see if it will sprout. If it doesn't sprout then the temperature was too high and you need to lower it until the grain sprouts. Cooking the bread at this precise temperature will conserve all its nutritive potency.

11. Undoubtedly the Angels of Heaven who made the golden grain that sprouts and grows can also make our daily bread.

12. For your holidays you can make a special bread sweetened

with raisins and honey and seasoned with anis and cinnamon to delight our guests.
13. This is the bread that your Celestial Father and your Earthly Mother provide for your dining table responding to your supplication and prayer, "Our Father who art in heaven, give us this day our daily bread."
14. This bread is the manna from heaven because it is known by the Angels of Heaven and is a living bread, a complete food because the heat of the sun didn't snatch away the subtle and delicate ingredients that remain intact, alive and active giving strength, vigor and health and also a long life to the sons and daughters who partake of this whole grain bread, whole because it contains all the ingredients and nutritional factors that the human body needs.
15. This is the same bread that kept Methuselah strong for so many hundreds of years (969) and the same bread that fed your parents in their exodus from Egypt and the same bread that gave tremendous strength to thousands of slaves who dragged and lifted huge stone blocks to construct the pyramids.
Here are the Editorial Notes explaining why Dr. Johnny Lovewisdom did not translate the Spanish version exactly as it was published. Editorial Notes: Those who have not received the True Initiation of John, the Illumined Initiator, still being bread-lovers do their utmost to censor and pervert all the Johanine Scriptures and his Initiation. John neither ate meat, or bread, drank wine, or preached doctrines advocating grains or bread for food. The Aramaic Peshitta N.T. originals help in interpreting the true teachings: As in Matthew 13:31,32 where it speaks of the grain of mustard seed, the word for seed is used for any plant grown as a crop, such as grain, vegetables, etc., many of our vegetables being of the mustard family. Whether one uses wheat or grains or vegetable seeds depends on the climate one lives in, what seed is available and prefers for food. In cold Canadian, Siberian, etc. climates, wheat grass, buckwheat lettuce, sunflower greens, tender pea vines, etc. give a quick garden within a protected warm room with windows. In a warm tropical or summer climate one never needs to use grosser grain foods that destroy the soil, since so many tender vegetables adapt so easily. The baking of bread must be replaced by the photosynthesis of green plants which give chlorophyll, or iron and other minerals in nutritional needs. If one resorts to drying greens this must be

done in a dark room or bags since sunshine destroys chlorophyll. Another key in translating that a bread-eater's psychology misses in this chapter is that of the Aramaic word used here for sprouting or the springing up in growth of a plant which is identical to the Mark IV parable of the sower indicating that seed that fell on stony ground and lacking earth, the seed could not take root, withered and died, so that one must use earth to plant. Otherwise, just soaking wheat and sprouting, or even growing a vegetable from grain or other seed in a pan without earth, is like the farmer who plants cooked grain expecting something from unfruitful conditions like fools. The burning sun can be deadly to living tissue, causing cancer, sun-stroke, etc. in humans, or it can burn papayas, pineapple, and other fruits and vegetables while on the growing plant so they rot rather than ripen. Off the plant, in warm climates you can cook vegetables and fruits in the hot midday sun. It matters not whether one scalds, scorches, or burns, it kills the living plant tissue which withers and dies rendering such food to be dead just as much as when it is cooked on a stove or oven. A blade of grass grown from wheat, or an herb, or green leafy vegetable is the same word as is the case with Mt. 13:26, Mk. 6:39 and Heb. 6:7 in Aramaic. Secular clergy and others were able to pervert John's Initiation by putting the punctuation in the wrong places and using double meanings of some words, contrary to John's teaching against the use of grains and the use of fire to cook, living from that which nature provided freely.

    The profane, secular priest soon elaborated ceremonies of the Holy Mass, using bread and wine, against the will of the real Establisher and Initiator. At the Last Supper, in the Johannine Initiation, the allegory must refer to wine fruit or grape juice, and living bread meaning succulent vegetable, fruit or plant yielding a fount of living water springing up into Life Everlasting, referring to God's Paradisian Plan in Genesis and for the Kingdom of Heaven on earth. Living Water was the secret Universal Alkahest or Solvent that Alchemists sought to obtain Life Everlasting, or the Eternal Living Fire fed on Living Water, shedding the Living Light that would uplift all mankind and beings on earth beyond suffering in shackles of misery. In the True Initiation of John, one becomes a Son of God, or the "Son of the sun of the Sun, since the sun was only a lens thru which the Light and the Source of all Life and Omnipotence passes from the Center of the Cosmos.

Simon Magus remained with a split personality of the flesh fighting his spirit within his mind, so while holding some of John's spiritual doctrines of a blood-free sacrifice adopted in Church Mass, yet he allowed for popular patronage by permitting bread and wine. As seen in the Gospel of Paul in his Epistles he is ever saying that he is justified by spirit and not the Law of God, by grace and because he is an Apostle, Minister, etc. just as Christian clergy imitated in Church doctrines.

Publisher's Note: Sprouted grain bread is useful as part of a systematic, detoxifying, transition diet leading toward a mucuslean or mucusless diet of fruit, plus herbs as needed; lettuce, spinach, celery, carrot, parsley, basil etc. Sprouted bread, cooked brown rice, cooked potatoes and rye crisp bread are transition foods and not ideal. The same holds true for raw milk and cultured raw milk products. Grains and raw milk products help slow down the elimination process. The reason we can deduce this is because in the text of the *God Spell* it says that Moses' law on diet was superseded by the new law given in the *God Spell*. Since raw milk products and sprouted grains are mucus forming and therefore eventually disease producing, they are not ideal foods, yet useful in slowly detoxifying the body. Consult *The Healing Transition Diet* in the appendix of *The Buddhist Essene Gospel of Jesus* for more information.

CHAPTER XXXV (1-26)

Once the Healer's commentary ceased, one of the listeners still could not fathom its depth of meaning so as to come up with the question: "Why is it bad to eat bread, or do you blame stomach aches, indigestion and difficulty to evacuate the bowels as being due to bread eating?"

The Savior continued, "All this is due to many causes. The principal cause is that people do not know what they suffer from. The Living Food I have been advocating, certainly does not cause the pain and trouble when dead bread is eaten with it, because Living Foods contain all the ingredients necessary for good digestion, evacuation and health. Let us imagine we are watching the food as it goes thru the body's digestive organs.

In the mouth food is chewed with the teeth. You should slowly masticate your food mixing it well with the saliva till the food becomes wholly (simply) Living Water, so one can fully enjoy the satisfaction of one's appetite. As one chews, the Living Food turns more and more into Living Liquid, so it begins to flow down the throat into the stomach, where the food begins to flow down the throat into the stomach, where the food begins digestion, then meets with the bloodstream, giving blood its vital force. The more we chew our food in the mouth making it a Living Liquid, the easier it is for it to be transformed into the Life Stream of our body. One should never gulp food down without chewing it, turning it into a liquid similar to saliva, to avoid stomach trouble, and to assure one that one will not have other digestive troubles, and to get the full benefit every mouthful provides. Even the soft foods like ripened fruits and clabber must be mixed well with the saliva, fully tasting and gaining full satisfaction, before allowing it to be swallowed, to give health and strength. Then, travelling from the stomach to the intestines, this liquid food shall return to a soft mass, after the Living Liquid is absorbed and the fiber contained sweeps out the old residues of past meals from the intestinal tube, allowing for full assimilation and evacuation without troubles.

When you eat baked bread, especially if the outer covering of the grain is removed, this will cause a pasty mass to be formed in the intestines, which sticks to the walls of the digestive tube, gathering unused waste matter from past meals causing the intestine to get bigger and bigger, obstructing passage, no matter how hard one tries to move the bowels. This in turn produces fermentation and decay in the masses retained, giving gas, digestive ailments, pain and suffering constipation.

Moreover, the fiber in Living Food has a very important part in the process since it enables food to travel easier thru the intestines because the fiber acts like a broom, sweeping, brushing, scrubbing, pushing and cleaning out the intestinal passage effectively, leaving them free from food waste, without sticking and clogging therein. All of this is very necessary for, not only having normal and undelayed evacuation of the bowels, but for a clean and pure blood stream.

Also, the fiber in food also stimulates the production of a waxy or oily surface to the mass of food waste, to lubricate or prevent adherence so the wastes do not stick to the intestinal walls, allowing for their easy evacuation. This is like an anointing balsam that purifies, heals and prevents rotting putrification so as to cause the healing of injuries, irritation, ulceration and formation of hemorrhoids. Often this waxy substance covering our foods (uncooked fruits and vegetables) is also a necessary purifying and appetizing essence (enzymes) required to produce the mouth-watering flow of saliva, assuring good digestion, appetite and a clean breath in the mouth. The fiber in food gently scrubs the teeth without hurting their surface, preventing cavities, rotting of foods further in the intestines causing intestinal fever and other internal fevers. The waxy, or oily coverings contain a purifying essence that prevents stinking, fetid or evil smelling bowel evacuations.

If one has evil smelling evacuations, it is a sure sign that where they came from,- the digestive tract,- is also in disorder and evil-smelling, in fermentation and putrification, due to the unused, improper and incompatible food substances that one eats, or does not chew well in good food. This endangers one's health, poisoning the blood with internal toxic waste putrification causing irritation, ulcers, tumors, hemorrhoids and other ailments.

Perhaps you have observed how water fowl, the swans, geese and others, oil or wax their feathers with an oil that is secreted by a gland which prevents their feathers from getting wet or causing mud to adhere to them, even if they go into dirty and muddy swamps, always remaining immaculately clean. In the same way the wax or oily essence contained in the covering or peel of whole living foods, internally anoints one's digestive tract preventing the adherence of food wastes and filth, so that it will always remain clean so that the living liquid nourishment of living food can be absorbed thru the membranes into the bloodstream, keeping the blood immaculately pure, which is the basic foundation for maintaining perfect health.

Editorial Notes: It was recorded that John abhorred the sight of shambles where the flesh of sacrificed animals was sold, which makes evident that he understood the great living intelligence with which each part of the digestive tract functioned changing the Living Liquids of grass or other foods that animals and man eats into the living bloodstream, and thus could not see how brute men, especially theological doctors at the Temple of Jerusalem, etc., could ignor such Omniscient Works of God, worthy of beholding reverence, sacrificed for flesh to satisfy the lust of their bellies. Even modern myopic bible critics talk glibly of pious petty theories, speaking of these holy men as being rustic ignoramuses, not realizing that they had been trained at the Carmelite Colleges of the Essenes, and lived practical, useful lives teaching others up to advanced ages. Living Longer lives, the ancients developed greater, more complete and more mature perspectives as compared to hasty faddist short-thinking solutions of today's overnight scientific marvels. John himself lived beyond the century mark. St. Irenaeus (192 A.D.), on the authority of Polycarp who had it from St. John himself and all the old people of Asia, that the Savior was not crucified, had said, "As the chief part of 30 years belongs to youth, and everyone will confess him such till 40 years, but from the 40th to the 50th year he declines into old age, which our Lord having attained, he taught us the Gospel and all the Elders who, in Asia assembled with JOHN, the disciple of the Lord, testify and as John himself taught them. And he remained with them till the time of Trajan" (who ruled till 117). The Koran also states that, "Yet they slew not Jesus Christ, neither crucify him, but he was represented by one in his likeness". The evidence from those authoritative sources and others, shows not only that an allegorical interpretation of the N.T. Bible is justified, but also that the chief hero was telescoped into appearing to be 3 or more characters to the Uninitiated reader (as even advanced critics still remain): Our Lord Jesus Christ of Christians is only the title of John, the Establisher-Initiator of his Church, while John, the Apostle Beloved of Christ, is still the same person thru whom the Lord speaks God's revelations. Today priests continue the same practice in that outside the alter and pulpit they speak as ordinary people, but thereon they officiate as the Lord Christ incarnate, in other words a vicar of Christ. Our mission on earth in the Apostolate of the laity, or priestly power of all humans, is to be the Lord God in action, which most people are so far removed from being that they cannot imagine themselves as being or doing in practice. Matthew 27:32, Mark 15:21, Luke 23:26 all state that Simon of Cyrene's time (a Galilean who was a Zealot, Josephus said was crucified) took Christ's (John's) place in the crucifixion. In John 19:15 it specifically uses the word used to indicate both EXALT and Crucify so as to conceal the real meaning when Pilate said, "Shall I crucify your king?", the Jews demanding his crucifixion. So they took Simon of Galilee and crucified him as "The King of the Jews" in mockery of their unjust demands. Both Pilate and Herod had been enemies but because they agreed as to finding no fault with John, or "Jesus" himself, and became united in the mystic knowledge of John's Initiation, they all became fraternal friends, which also became the day the Gnostic Christians or Followers of John and all the Essenes abandoned the Jews to their self-made fate. Many Gnostics condemned the Jewish doctrine, save a few groups of Essenes unaware of the mystic secret. All this was hidden under allegories about the resurrection of John and Jesus as they remained concealed under new titles. Thus John, as founder of the Mandaeans, in Samaria he was known as Manaendros, or Manaen of Antioch, and Cerinthus or Merinthus of Ephesus. Manaen of Antioch described as the foster brother of Herod confirms the Gnostic fraternal relationship among those who could not bear the "eye for eye, tooth for tooth" dogma of hate fostered by the synagogue, and the Essenes continued in Buddhist doctrines in Antiochian, Ephesian and Greek Pythagorean as well as Alexandrian Circles but with later sanctions as being "Gnostics" by the Roman Church after Constantine in the 4th century.

Returning to the testimony of this chapter, as to the Inner Sanctuary Gnostic Teaching, not only is there acknowledgement of an external "Exoteric" baptism and anointing of the body, but True Initiates of John had to comply with the Esoteric deeper INNER BAPTISM of Living Water and INNER ANOINTING of the Living Chrism, that only Living Food cast down from Heaven provide. The vibration, aura, smell, elimination and other tell-tale signs confirm the Inner Initiation of Gnostic Christians of St. John. "Meat" and "Bread" in Aramaic texts, one must realize had no word for food and thus they mean food. Moreover, to become part of the Anointed Savior's Mystical body and blood of Christ, they can say "I am the Living Bread cast down from Heaven, If any man eat of this bread, he shall live forever, and the bread I give is my flesh for the life of mankind." Other bread is death, and whenever he spoke of food you must know it is LIVING FOOD and Living Water that he speaks of, or it is not of him, neither Living or the Chrism of the Anointed. In Aramaic the word for "whole" also means simple and guileless, as in Mt. 10:16, Rom. 16:19, as is the frugal food of the poor, like the carob husks in which the peel or covering is eaten, which one may correspond with eating the peel on ripe bananas, papaya, apple, cucumbers, carrot, etc. which contain valuable minerals, enzymes and the Inner Chrism of the Initiate. (We find prudence is required as to thorny pineapple, citrus peels, etc. since one can only discover the Path of the LIVING WORD in experience, and not sharp delineations of words, dogmatic laws and polemies. The Golden Mean easily distinguishes the True Initiate, yet the uninitiated will find exception because they seek fault.

Thus, the followers of Simon, as the Rock "Petros" of the Faith of the Roman Church, and John, the Initiator, Manda or Gnostic Christian who knew, rather than holding to blind faith, separated into the Seven Churches of Asia, or Eastern Ecclesia and Western Papacy, with Inner and External teachings. What Christianity had on the surface differed from the deepest inner core like the Heavens and earth, so far and yet so near really, if one gets an inner perspective of the True Initiation.

CHAPTER XXXVI (1-37)

Then the Anointed Savior continued teaching them about making meals Sacred or Sanctifying their Eucharistic Table in their homes. First he told them, "NEVER EAT WITHOUT HUNGER. Do not sit at the Table until you are called by the Angel of Hunger. The feeling of hunger is produced by the cells involved with food assimilation, when they are free and ready for a new ration of food. When there is no appetite it means that these cells are still trying to digest a previous meal. If you eat in that case, you are provoking indigestion, stomachache and diarrhea.

When you gather at the Common Table in your homes, you should also do so contented, rejoicing and in good humor. Leave behind all thoughts that cause serious worry, because these are contagious and will sadden others around one, and the food eaten under such conditions becomes toxic. Your mind should emanate Love, forgiveness and beauty like the aromatic flowers with which you should decorate your common table. Again I repeat, never sit at the table unhappy, irritated and in bad humor, because these Satanic emotions decompose the blood, the digestive juices and poison one from within, which in extreme circumstances can cause paralysis within you or even sudden death.

Always bear in mind, that the Common Table is your ALTAR, and the place you eat your food is a Holy Sanctuary, where you actually prepare for the Transubstantiation of food and drink into the health, strength and Life of your blood and body. For this reason you should adorn the Holy Table (Holy-Mass in English or "mess table", Missa in Latin) like you do an Altar, with aromatic blossoms from your garden, and beautiful thoughts flowering in your hearts. Thus, in this auspicious environment (like, if not actually a Paradisian Garden), the Head of the Congregation shall start the silent ceremonial with blessing thanks for the food that never failingly is provided each day. With clean hands he takes part in the food in the sight of all those present establishing a solemn disposition. Once peace and calm is established thru-out the congregation, with the Head thanks is given to the Lord (the Holy Eucharist of Church ritual) spontaneously realized each day when correctly done.

As this is performed, with the head of the Table of those gathered, they participate in the transformation of living food into pure living blood that shall give health, peace and the Joy in Living, beside the Wisdom of good works, righteousness, justice, honesty, charity and love. However, in order that all these things come about, or that the Lord shall bless and consecrate our Living Food, and be Present at our Holy Table, there must be perfect harmony, mutual pardon, peace and love among the congregation, because the pure holy feelings of each one present elevates the joy and happiness of everyone which begets rejoicing in the Lord or the Spontaneity of the Divine Spiritual Presence.

Where there is Peace, Harmony and Love, there also is God, because God is Harmony, God is Peace and God is Love. In God's Presence we find his Angels, and among them also the Angel of Joy, who shall dwell and swell in your hearts with Rejoicing, Gladness and Happiness, and who give us intense Living Joy."

Then the Master Healer began to teach about the amount of food we should eat, saying, "Altho there may be many and much delicious food on your Table, eat only of a few kinds, and only the amount needed to satisfy hunger. One should seek the Attitude of Gratitude in the most precious habit of NOT EATING IN EXCESS, since it is the vice of Gluttony that makes one ill, and worse violates God's Commandments. It is advisable to measure a certain amount of food when eating, neither too little or too much, always in balance. One should eat neither a great amount, nor a great variety of kinds of food mixed together. One has to eat only a few kinds of food in one meal, because many kinds of distinct classes in general neither tolerate one another, nor can they even combine well. To the contrary, they may repel one another and cause disorder, warring with one another, giving one an upset stomach and internal pains. The root cause of the trouble is the fact that each kind of food has a determined and different time for digestion, being absorbed by the blood and used in the structural economy of one's body. When certain foods of rapid, easy digestion are thru digesting, they must pass from the stomach to the intestines, and consequently carry undigested foods of difficult slow absorption with them. This provokes fermentation and putrification in the intestines, causing swelling or fetid gases, ulcers, hemorrhoids, constipation and result in evacuations that are troublesome and evil smelling. All of this teaches one the valuable lesson coming from such disorders, which is that even the healthiest foods eaten together with other foods that need a different time to digest, can cause digestive ailments. To avoid this, one should eat one class of foods (fruits, or a vegetable meal) with only two or three kinds in a meal (carrots, greens and clabber plants in a meal) or what one knows to combine well by previous experience, giving no trouble.

The truth about these matters is that if you mix many foods together in one meal, eating your fill of them, it is quite probable that this mixture of foods will make you feel bad, because the intolerance of one kind, or incompatibility with another kind of antagonistic food, will decompose the whole concoction within your bowels.

So let not the vice of gluttony overcome you like the servant who was invited to eat at the Table of the Lord, and because he was an insatiable glutton he greedily devoured not only his own share of food but also that of all the others, becoming so full that he vomited all he had eaten. This blunder so displeased the Lord, that he was sent away from the table and never invited again. So one should never rapidly devour a meal. Eat very slowly, taking time to avoid acquiring excessive weight, a bulging belly, which is a bad example, against nature and a sign of illness, caused by excessive gluttony, which is VICIOUS EATING or LIVING TO EAT and NOT EATING TO LIVE. Do not eat like pagans who rapidly devour all they can, get drunk and defile their bodies with every abominable thing they can do.

Beside, eating one's food slowly, taking one's time, of only well chosen and adequate foods for one's well being, one will require less food, because your whole body is better nourished from the food that is well chewed and mixed with the saliva and slowly eaten. In turn, when food is rapidly gulped down, the body only makes little use of it, or absorbing less than half of it. The rest of it, being unusable, is cast out in evil smelling excrement. Chew each mouthful carefully with your teeth, slowly taking time to mix it well with saliva, until it becomes a Living Liquid so the Aquarian Angel may Transubstantiate it into Living Blood, that will be Pure, Vibrant with Health, Energy and Strength.

Editorial Notes: This Chapter on the Holy Eucharist seeks to bring out the Attitude of Gratitude that Spontaneously prevails at a Paradisian Meal when the partakers are Spiritually advanced, beyond the worldly mind with its maximum of exceeding in complaints, calumny and vexation, as well as God's Presence when Garden fruits become one's food and object of one's work. Idleness does not bring true Spontaneity of Joy and Thankfulness in Living. Perhaps one of the best and earliest records of the basic Christian principles, which today is lost in vain sanctimonious ceremony and outer ritual, is the Doctrine of the Twelve Apostles or "Didache". This is dated to have appeared about the year 90 A.D., being a Manual for Piety and not a ritual, and believed to be of the "Saints" (Christians) of the "Ecclesia" (Church) of Antioch. No one was to be permitted at the Holy Eucharistic Table but those who were Baptized in the Name of the Father, the Son and the Holy Spirit in LIVING WATER. The original words continue from John's Initiation, altho the meaning now given is far from the Essence of the Essene Purity or Living Gnosis. According to the Didache the "Our Father" was to be prayed 3 times a day by the Saints, at 9 AM, 12 and 3 PM, according to St. Clement of Alexandria, "altho the PERFECT CHRISTIAN, OR GNOSTIC, PRAYS ALL THE TIME", showing that the First Christians, or Gnostics, practiced or lived their Prayer, rather than make words replace being Love, or GOD IN ACTON IN OUR LIVES, feeling His Joy, Thanks and Charity toward all. Similar to the Didache, also this chapter warns against the false prophets who do not live by the Table Manners and Habits of Saints, greedily gulping down their food in excesses, ending in vomiting, gas and indigestion.

CHAPTER XXXVII (1-12)

Another factor that is necessary for good digestion and assimilation of food is deep breathing. Air is the MOST IMPORTANT FOOD. You can live many days without any food, but within a short period we can die for lack of air. So one should make a habit of breathing deeply always, because the Elemental Spirit (Angels, fairies, fays, fauns, elves, pixies, etc. found in myths, fables, traditions and poetry of all nations ancient and modern) of Air is as necessary for the digestion of food as air is needed for fire to burn fire-wood in the hearth. If one does not breathe well, digestion becomes difficult, so that we only use a SMALL PART OF THE FOOD WE EAT, and the rest is cast out into the privy, or worse if the wastes clog the intestines, enlargening one's abdomen or produce false fatness (edema).

So, remember that all the false stoutness that one has to carry around with one wherever one goes always, like a heavy load, from which one can never be free, unless one sticks to a strict dietetic discipline consisting of fasting, and eating only fruits and vegetables, which means a VITARIAN REGIMEN. It is commonly known that excessive weight is an obstacle in very many jobs, occupations and athletics. It shows the disadvantage that a fat or corpulent body has against a lean one. A beautiful body among humans does not consist in being stout, but rather in slender stature and lean of flesh. The less excess weight a person has, the more strength a person will have. One can do more, and one is the least worn out by prolonged mental and intellectual works.

My Beloved Disciples, you can do much good for the fat folk by advising them to fast, and partake of a VITARIAN DIETETICS, and helping them practice this Discipline, which is the only way one can take away excessive weight and give them a graceful figure as well as lean stature.

Editorial Notes: To some who read this translated originally Aramaic Scripture, it will seem preposterously coincidental that John the Baptist, or Jesus speaking thru him, would be using the very words and teachings that Johnny Lovewisdom has used or coined for naming his doctrine (Vitarian Diet, Vitalogical Sciences). However, until I had seen this Scripture and studied it in detail, I had not been so assured that I was the spiritual incarnation of John, and thus can account for the identical teaching, altho where other translators have failed (in the N.T. Bible, Szekely Version etc.), I have been able to supply the Aramaic correction in interpretation, to correspond identically with the Living Word of the Living God speaking from within at present. Thus, it was not necessary to use obsolete expressions of the first century when the message can be given in the required scientific language of our time. Many people have wondered why on our diet one gets so slender, not realizing that worldly foods of vicious and passionate excesses breed passionate corpulent flesh. Carnal foods give a carnal body and Carnal passions. Spiritualizing Dietetics gives birth to a New Race and New Age. We are literally burdened the least by the flesh, beside the vicious desires that obesity engenders. Without training, working at the typewriter and formerly growing my Paradise, I can easily lift my body weight chinning with my arms, or what most men of similar conditions find impossible due to superfluous flesh. Moreover, this Chapter brings out the importance of building lung capacity which so aided me in my early twenties climbing Andes mountain-sides, which accounts for good digestion, oxidation of body metabolic wastes, and resultant joyous entrancement with Life. Papius, who was a hearer of John among those resurrected from the dead by the Christ, claiming he, John, was alive still in Hadrian's time (117-138 A.D.), does not seem absurd to me, considering the obstacles John's Initiation removes from living longer.

CHAPTER XXXVIII (1-26)

Verily, verily, I say unto you, you are what you eat: Food characterizes the consumer, determines one's actions and how one reacts in everyday living. If you eat the flesh of animals, which are dead carcasses in a rapid state of decomposition and putrification, this also shall be your fate, beside animalizing one's character, because this flesh is impregnated with their bestial character or emotions of the dead animal. These lower evil emotions become one's nature, making one live like an animal without being aware of anything else. It is a sad, painful world, unworthy of humans, one's heart becomes callous, even hurting and killing others, becoming criminals, beside pessimists, selfish, stingy, materialists and atheists without God or Lawless. In turn, if one eats only Living Food, as do Vitarians, these foods will humanize one, give one a humanitarian Character, allowing one to ascend to higher levels of attainment, and even Spiritualize the consumer to become Divine in Nature, in which Happiness, Beauty and Love reign. This Higher Heavenly Sensitivity refines one's behavior so one becomes incapable and unworthy of hate, jealousy, insults, and hurting or killing anything. All one's actions become Noble, one becomes charitable, honest, righteous and truthful, a model citizen, working to help others selflessly, pacifists, having Faith in God and obeying His Laws, in a word,- SPIRITUAL. Such is the radical and decisive nature of the influence and power of the food we consume on the character and behavior.

However, even if one eats only Living Food, one can EAT WRONG, if one does not know HOW TO EAT! This is why it is especially important to learn about Right Eating. One needs to know one is eating correctly, which is EATING TO LIVE, and not just LIVING TO EAT. Be not the friend of Gluttony. Be FRUGAL in diet. Never eat till your stomach is too full to eat more. The Golden Rule in Dietetics is to stop eating while one still has a good appetite for more. On this Vitarian Diet you may eat three times a day if one desires,- at sunrise, midday and sunset. One should NEVER eat one mouthful outside these times, because this shows one has a vicious habit of "snacking" all the time. Eating continually, or between meals, does not allow one to feel well, because it interferes with the digestion of the previous meal, giving digestive disorders. Moreover, beside disorderly eating courting disorder one is living in Gluttony, which the Divine Law severely punishes.

However, one should eat only twice a day for the best of health, which means going without breakfast. The final goal in dietetics is the ideal of eating only once a day, when the sun is at its zenith. However, if one has indigestion or a stomach ache or a headache or does not have an appetite, one should NOT eat any more meals, fasting until one is ready to eat again with a good appetite. Also, to overcome digestive disorders one can partake only of the purest Living Water, which may be found in the form of Lime or Lemon juice: sour limes or lemons are best, altho sweet limes or lemons are very good too (but they contain sugars). Such juices cleanse and refresh the digestive tract, altho the best healing method is to live exclusively from the fragrance of flowers and tree blossoms. A feverish stomach or any kind of internal fever responds well to partaking of such Living Water treatment, because fire is quenched with water.

Aside from such Living Water, I prescribe partaking of NO OTHER SUBSTANCE to heal the stomach (or other ailments), because the HEALER WITHIN you knows how and what Healing Agent, that of itself, make one well again. Any other remedy that mercenary medicine men prescribe is erroneous, and only destroys the healing action of the OMNISCIENT INTERNAL HEALER (SAVIOR) within one. You may not be able to see this Inner Healer within your body, and within everyone, but by his works you know how wonderfully he heals your injuries. The Vitarian Regimen, along with fasting, instead of making one weaker, gives one strength, insuring one of sound health and longevity. The Heavenly Father, who is the Author of the Human Body, knows perfectly well how many meals and how much food one needs to maintain health in the physical, mental and spiritual being of everyone of us. To be able to do this, one should eat only the fruits and vegetables in season of one's particular environment, both in accord to climate and time of year, to derive the most benefit from them.

EDITORIAL NOTES: Water from springs, streams, wells and earth sources, not only is dead water, but contains salt, iron oxide (rust), limestone and other inorganic minerals which accumulate in human cell tissues making older people's bodies lack the elastic, flexible qualities of youth, hardening arteries, stiffening joints, making bones brittle so they break easily. Distilled water is still dead water beside an unstable chemical causing unpredictable changes to better or worse. Dead inorganic water deposits itself in the body, taking 3 weeks or more to eliminate, radioactively tagged molecules have shown. In turn, living water, such as found in limes and lemons contain 97.6 % water in a living plant substance with enzymes and vitamins, which include living organic lime and other minerals we need to restore balance, and yet lacking food calories they act as cellular cleansers or purifiers, healthwise. One needs no water for short fasts, which makes them doubly effective as "dry fasts" and for longer periods one can use this citrus Living Water without food calories. It is a symbolic and literal truth that the long thorned fruits, especially ungrafted citrus, thorny pineapples, etc. contain the FLAMING SWORD guarding the path to the tree of Life in Paradise, and lacking food calories, seem designated to duties related to purification during fasting and prayer, or "morning and Sunday rest fruits".

A 7 year University course can only get one started EATING RIGHT, since I have spent 7 times 7 years working at its problems, learning still each day. Yet in the beginning it seemed so simple. Leaving home, going to wilds or jungle seemed like all there was to it. The wilds have fruit once a year requiring winter hibernation, and the jungle had none to speak of, until man plants mango-forests, banana plantations, and the like. Buddha spent 6 years living in wilds till he was unable to stand erect becoming a skeleton, and a mango diet will make one a skeleton. I experienced the untoward effects of tropical jungle life in Ecuador, finding only dense impassable forest without fruits, so going to live in a cacao grove, where I had avocados and bananas in abundance, doing worse. Plantains, the only banana I had an appetite for, is for baking like "the bread of the tropics", physic one, and bananas and avocados I have classed as worst, near nuts and seeds of fruit which I consider the FORBIDDEN FRUITS of Paradise. Fig leaves were really banana leaves, since plantains are named "musa Paradisiaca" due to this fact. Unable to breathe the densely humid hot jungle air of jungles, toxic from gases of rotting vegetation, I became so weak, that I could hardly stand up, let alone climb avocado trees. Plenty of ripe ones fall to the ground which one can share with hogs that root out jungle growth, but also carry all kinds of parasites, ascarid intestinal worms, amoebic dysentery, etc. In a short time my body was down to a 6 foot 4 inch skeleton from dysentery weighing 97 lbs. Frightened by a heart attack, I came to my senses and fled to high mountains where I put on 25 lbs. in 6 weeks, and 10 lbs. each month till I was 205 lbs. just eating vegetables, since food could be oxidized in the rare mt. air giving health. But after gardening at two locations, I was again tempted to try a higher jungle altitude, but only to come down with malaria, skin ulcers, etc. Then back to the top of the Andes at the crater lake Quilotoa, which was nice, but I despaired with 20 year wait ahead to see if fruits would produce enough for my needs. Abandoning it to run back to California, I only jumped into a worse hell; plenty of fruit everywhere but every bit poisoned. Weed-killers, pesticides, fertilizers and preservatives on fruits and vegetables destroyed the liver and kidney function and paralysis set in, ending up as human trash in a State Hospital "Snake Pit", against my own will, to receive a barrage of antibiotics, worsening the paralysis, neurosis, and finally the balance mechanism needed for walking was lost. Once rescued by kind friends, I fled to Ecuador to find now it is likewise plagued by chemical pesticide farming. One cannot dream such things away!

The Baptism or Initiation of John is no longer practical, no civilized person is able to adapt to such a life, no longer are liveable places found where one can live freely from what grows of itself. Newspapers tell us that, "Millions of Americans have been eating carrots heavily contaminated with endrine, aldrin or deldrin, this group of deadly poisons is incriminated as the cause of kidney, liver and heart disease. Carrots absorb unusually large quantities of dangerous pesticides. Excessive residues of toxaphene or endrine are found on leafy vegetables such as cabbages, parsley, cauliflower, broccoli, etc. 70% of the produce on the market today is coated with dangerous wax, paraffin, that never leaves the body after it is consumed, responsible for cancer and other ailments." And so on endlessly, with no stop in sight.

But, let us suppose you know all this, and do succeed in finding a place to grow your own food. Yet, because one has been poisoned by food in the past, now the new life without poison may be unbearable at times. One will get spasms, numbing, and neurosis trying to fast or living on pure liquids, since the fat of the body yields back toxins when used. After your teeth are formed, damage done, is hard to undo, and excess sweet fruit destroys enamel. Often the return to nature may create one's own POLLUTION PROBLEM WITHIN, so one can live neither with others, nor with oneself. One has to dodge from out under the stars, into outside shelters. In the Andes there is continual field and volcanic dust in the air, so rain water turns muddy, and if one does not use vegetable soap to wash the hair occasionally, the pretty blond hair of northerners will create a cloud of dust all around one every time one moves the head, and one cannot stand stuffy enclosures. Worse, one may lack oxidation of food wastes, not breathing well, eat wrong foods together at wrong times, the wrong way, lacking food metabolism, so that the intestines produce methane, sulphurous and other gases so stinky and toxic that neither alone, nor with others, can one live within walls. Tiny vermin can invade the hair and clothing making one unwanted in people's homes. Just cooking green vegetables drains out the body's calcium supply. WRONG EATING is a dangerous weapon!

CHAPTER XXXIX (1-7)

One should work from sunrise to sunset six days of the week, because WORK IS THE GREATEST DUTY OF MAN, the Divine Observance of God's Presence, and the BEST TEACHER FOR

MASTERY IN LIFE. During these days one should partake exclusively of the VITARIAN Diet. However, on the seventh day, one shall rest, consecrating it to the Heavenly Father completely by Fasting, or partaking only of Living Water in its purest form (limes, etc.). This seventh day, along with fasting, one should devote to Spiritual Prayer, or Meditation, Studying the Sacred Scriptures and other Spiritual works, and this New Age Teaching... In this way you shall be partaking exclusively of Spiritual Food the Seventh Day, for not only from (material) food liveth man, but from every Word of the Heavenly Father.

If it is at all possible, go out into sylvan solitudes or the desert on that seventh day, away from the hustle and bustle of worldlings, to give Praise to the Lord, Fast and Contemplate, and be alone with the Heavenly Angels of Sunshine, Air, Water and especially the Angels of Joy and Fasting. This is the Path of Attainment by which the Divine Angels prepare one for the death of self, for rebirth in the Heavenly Kingdom or Realm of Life Everlasting in God's Presence.

CHAPTER XL (1-7)

If you have worked hard at your work all day, after sunset you shall be tired and need to rest. Then the Heavenly Father shall send you the Angel of Sleep, who shall replenish your strength, and give you rest as you sleep. To be able to sleep during the night, you must not sleep during the day, because the day is for work and the night is for rest. Once your body is well rested and peaceful, your soul will become able to leave your body to visit the Heavenly Kingdom, where the Heavenly Powers (Spiritual Beings, Angels, Gods, etc. same word in Aramaic) shall receive you lovingly, teach you Higher Wisdom, and the Mysteries of the Higher Spiritual Realms.

Only those who have complied with the Commandments of Mother Nature will be fully able to awaken and become distinctly aware of the wonders of the Heavenly Realm. Once you are able to remain awakened or conscious in the Spiritual Kingdom within you, shall you be blessed with the Greater Spiritual Activity in Omnipotent Life Potential working in the Will of God. Then, each day will greet one with increased Joy in Living, because overcoming one's burdens in the sensual plane, one's work conforms to Truth and Spirit every moment of that day and always.

Editorial notes: Generally people live on the lower emotional plane, dreaming in the animalistic pleasure or pain attractions they create by thoughts, but meditation on the Higher Planes in time actually gives into Life therein. One's dreams become symbolic, illumining one's path. Finally, after receiving Higher Spiritual Initiations, one no longer remains unconscious, sleeping most of the night dwelling on the astral desire plane. The Higher Initiate sleeps very little, spending 20 hours more or less on the Higher Super-Conscious Realms out of 24, since Juicy fruits, succulent vegetables and clabber are directly assimilable, and 4 hours is all the rest required. The Elders of the HIGHER HEAVENLY HIERARCHY on earth (Great White Lodge of Gurus) who are cleansed receiving all the Higher Initiations, the Inner Baptisms of Living Water, Spiritual Anointing use the morning hours of each night to guide those who are ready to progress rapidly on the Higher Realms and their New Age application. Sensual folk find escape, either sleeping and dreaming while the body struggles with unnatural food burdens, or seek escape with narcotics, smoking and drinking and patronizing night life establishments, if not worse drugs.

CHAPTER XLI (1-9)

Now, the Savior, speaking thru John, spoke especially to those under his leadership, saying, "Beloved Disciples, you who aspire to become Apostles of the Healing God Spell, (Physician-Priests), must always teach thru your Living Example. You should never allow yourselves to become victims of mind bending drugs of any kind, much less narcotics and alcoholic drinks. The Apostles of the Healing Spiritual Entrancement shall abstain from all drinks and stupefacient drugs, no matter what the occasion. They shall only partake of pure Living Water, whenever they assemble and give praise to God. Just as it is most difficult to straighten a crooked tree which has grown old, so also it is trying to convert an old chronic alcoholic. But you can avoid difficulty by planting the tree with care from the seed, so the roots grow deep, straight down and the trunk straight up with strong guiding stakes to protect it from growing crooked. Likewise, in order that mankind shall not entirely turn to drinking and drug addiction and the crooked path going from one pleasure to another, you must become the Guiding Stakes, The Elder, Masters or Teachers, teaching the young folk thru selfless service by your LIVING EXAMPLE, in not letting any such corrupting influence completely swallow mankind. Then as the children and youth mature into men and women of mankind, they shall ever remember your exemplary teachings, and continue to teach their young folk, in turn, becoming their guiding stakes. Only by this Everlasting Self-Vigilant Path shall we uproot these terrible vices from this present world, and establish the Disciplined, Abstinent, Healthy, Powerful and Happy New Race.

CHAPTER XLII (1-18)

You who aspire to become the Apostles of the Healing God Spell, shall ever be the BRAVE GUIDES, who, without truce or compromise, shall untiringly combat the evil vices that accompany alcoholism. By this I mean, opposing such mind bending vices as using any kind of dope, opium, tobacco, gambling, prostitution, and many more, because such evil habits bring the downfall and ruin of man in his wearisome ascension climbing up to the snow-capped Heights of Perfection required to purify and guide mankind from its defects. The pioneers to the Heights of Illumination are ever being attacked on their path upward by these loathsome bandits who often leave their victims beaten and mortally wounded by the wayside. Here, I am not referring to the flesh and blood bandits, but even more so to one's own evil habits, harbored within one's soul, often in subtle forms, which likewise may catch one unaware, leaving one beaten by the wayside, worse than by such marauders.

Your work as GOOD SAMARITANS shall come to the rescue of these brave Pilgrims abandoned on the wayside of this Road in Life. Help them overcome their moral and physical suffering, give them a helping hand in support so they can get to a sheltered place where regeneration shall be possible. One of the places that one finds many of these victims abandoned by the wayside in everyday life is in the prisons, where you may help by working in the regeneration of these deserted moral victims.

The First Teaching they need to learn is that THERE IS NO PERFECT CRIME, meaning there is no crime without Punishment. These victims should know that they too have a Higher Master Teacher, or Tutelary Spirit, that is invisibly watching over one, unknown, but allowing for reward in one's good works, and punishing one's evil ones. Just as soon as these shackled victims begin planning new violations, they are discovered, which they need to know before they continue such mental paths, since their own thoughts betray them. Each new thought at its very moment of conception is automatically being recorded or engraved in the LIVING ARCHIVES of Natural Genetic Memory where one's Tutelary Master arranged for one's future as to such crooked intentions.

This is because the Life we live is a SCHOOL OF EXPERIENCE, in which one profits by one's downfalls. The Invisible Guiding Teacher allows one to realize one's evil intentions, which even in one's perversity teach one the Lessons of Life. They are what cause one to undergo all kinds of bitter experiences, punishments and warnings, to eventually get so tired and weary in such a vicious path, that one finally surrenders, repents and rectifies one's conscience, at the same time he arranges Justice to trap one, giving one time at a reformatory. This is why we have prisons, so the shackled victims can be forced to reform and tire of sin. Like the prodigal son learned, by forced work one learns to earn an honest living so as to avoid future detention. Again we see how the Heavenly Father tenderly loves his sons and daughters and has real compassion for those who fall. He does not want to destroy or kill anyone: He only wants to give one ANOTHER CHANCE in Life to make straight one's path, reform, regenerate and learn how to become useful members of Mankind. (end of scripture) This is the end of the scripture as translated by Dr. Johnny Lovewisdom. The publisher will here include Chapter 41, 45, 46 and part of 30 (table salt), translated from the Spanish language version because these chapters were not translated. Chapter 41:
1. In the New Spiritual Age, that has now begun, the death penalty will be abolished and replaced by the sentence of mandatory regeneration of the delinquent, because the death sentence opposes the supreme law of "Thou shall not kill" because only God has the right to take away life.
2. The death sentence translates into hate your neighbor through cruel vengeance in applying the hateful penalty of an eye for an eye and a tooth for a tooth.
3. The law of hate is outdated and is now replaced by the Law of love, the highest law in the world (Universe) because it is this law that makes possible your existence. This Law motivates you to serve everyone without looking at who it is, like the Good

Samaritan who felt sorry for the injured person lying on the roadside. The law of love means compassion, pity and pardon, that the sick will find health and the fallen will rise up again, the ignorant will be instructed, educated and disciplined, teaching them a profession so they can make a living honorable through their own work.

4. Compulsory regeneration will miraculously empty the prisons, reduce the number of judges and police officers and reduce the ignorance in the lowest social spheres, elevating their cultural level.

5. The truly regenerated criminal generally is born in their next reincarnation as an honest, decent, respected, hard working citizen who has an immense wealth of practical knowledge, are creators of industries, arts and trades. They are a positive factor in the general progress of society.

6. By comparison, for each criminal that is not regenerated and condemned to death, another criminal will be born in the next life with other reborn criminals and they will fill the prisons, the gambling halls, the whorehouses, the crackhouses, the insane asylums etc. They are a major factor in the backsliding of society in general.

7. By way of the mistaken justice of the death penalty the crime in the world will be artificially increased, filling our streets with bad citizens and our prisons with prisoners freezing social progress in its tracks.

8. The judge that condemns a human being to death will receive a valuable lesson because giving a fatal sentence to a prisoner will sentence that very judge to being the parent of that criminal in the next life.

9. Now, being his own child the judge will do all that he can to help the child progress, educating him, teaching him until finally after so much sacrifice the child is converted into a useful member of society, respectable and good, someone who contributes to the social and economic well-being of the country.

10. This will serve to teach the former judge that if they ever are again in such an important position they need to judge as if the accused was his own child and sentence them to mandatory regeneration and not to death, because only in this way will they not reincarnate in a retarded fashion, and they will be regenerated in this very life which will further their evolution.

Chapter 45: Begins on the next page.

1. To end these lessons I see that I have not mentioned the highest virtue of Purity and I am referring to Sexual Purity.
2. Procreation is a Supreme Law of Life put in place by the Celestial Father to perpetuate the human race. Procreation is a sacred, sublime act that must be respected and executed with immaculate purity.
3. Executing the act of procreation as God commands it, under the most scrupulous purity, the parents assure themselves of a prize from the Celestial Father and that is a sound and outstanding descendency. The most advanced souls who are waiting on the other side are obliged to return to the earth to continue their education; these same souls seek pure bodies to incarnate in and prefer naturally those bodies produced by parents of immaculate sexual purity. Only this will ensure the birth of beautiful children with slender bodies and gifted with a wholesome health and above average intelligence of notable spiritual and moral qualities.
4. Children from such a pure birth the Celestial Father watches over and pours down His blessings and good fortune which will assure a bright future for these children and will constitute the greatest happiness of their parents.
5. To achieve a birth of such optimum conditions, the parents before performing the sexual act must purify and strengthen their bodies. This is achieved before anything by an adequate diet.
6. The proper food for parents who are about to conceive a child is fruit and vegetable based, raw vegetarian diet. This because only in a raw state do vegetables conserver all their vital force. They should avoid all meat and alcoholic beverages and above all give up all tobacco because these vices excite the lower instincts of men making them commit fornication. On the other hand raw vegetarianism awakens the higher faculties, the Divine in the man inducing him to the a pure sexual life.
7. The immense importance of raw food vegetarianism for the procreation of extraordinary children is revealed in the Sacred Bible where it mentions the birth of Samson. The mother of Samson was visited by a Divine messenger announcing that she will have a very wise son and who will also be the strongest physically who ever lived. But there was a demand that the future mother must comply with and that was that she only eat raw vegetarian food and that her only drink will be pure water.

She must eliminate all meat and alcoholic beverages. She complied with these rules and the son that was born was so strong and robust that at 14 years of age he fought a lion that attacked him and killed it with his bare hands. Later in his life he fought the Philistines who attacked and he defeated and killed all of them. Due to his extraordinary intelligence he was elected judge and king of the Israelites.

8. If parents wish to have such extraordinary children, they need to imitate the parents of Samson. Before they engage in the procreative act they need to go on a strict regimen for at least three months before conception and the mother must continue the regimen throughout the pregnancy and breast feeding so that the son will partake of the food of the mother. During the three months prior to conception the couple must live a pure, calm life breathing the pure air of the country or the seashore. I repeat that no meat should be eaten, nor alcoholic drinks drunk, nor cigarettes smoked and their food should only be raw vegetarian meals and pure water, exercising, breathing pure air and sunbathing.

9. Only in this way, imitating this couple, and before all else the example of this magnificent mother that God used as the model for mothers of all times. This couple can rest assured in the birth of a robust child that could be the next Samson.

Chapter 46   (Note: Some are "called" to have children and some are not.)

1. Procreation in its maximum purity is practiced by the animals such as the deer, horses, camels, elephants etc., because the male animal only seeks the female and the female the male when they are in heat and apart from this time they refuse all sexual relations even though they live together in brotherly harmony.

2. When human beings begin to follow this Natural Law that the animals respect so rigorously, then they will have reached the highest grade of civilization and culture.

3. But... when the sex act degenerates into a vice, a mere sensual pleasure, then it is no longer called procreation... it is fornication, which means the lowest relaxation of the most sacred function of procreation.

4. But... when the sex act degenerates to the most profound abysm of sodomy (homosexuality), and all means of regeneration have failed then imminent justice condemns such depraved, incorrigibles to be burned alive, like the inhabitants of Sodom, Gomorrah, Zeboyim and Admahs. These cities were swept by the

divine broom into the garbage so that they could be burned in one trash heap, one bonfire.

5. Nonetheless... such depraved individuals can save themselves from being burned alive if they repent in time with their whole heart and begin to energetically battle their terrible vice in order to uproot it completely from their brain and heart. From there they need to vehemently reject all those thought and emotions that invite the vice. In this Titanic fight the Sodomites can serve to show that the long fast, raw vegetarianism and above all prayer or asking help from heaven are the most effective weapons.

6. Because it is true that the Supreme goal of man on earth is to reach the highest summit of purity, dignity and culture, it is also true that sodomy is the opposite point or in other words the lowest abysm of impurity, indignity and culturelessness.

7. For this reason the Mother Earth refuses to accept the ashes of such depraved individuals, opening at the scene of the crime a huge abysm that is full of putrid, salty waters that kill all beings or germs that are alive, so that no life can prosper in those waters, for which reason this dark lake is called the Dead Sea, which serves to always remind the cities that Sodomy will exterminate them until the most absolute sterility is realized.

Publisher's Note: In the following verses you will note that a modern day addition was made to the original scripture. Emil Mogner translated the Aramaic original into German in 1899 and he must have added the following verses since it mentions the German ship Neptune and the year 1903, which is just 4 years after 1899 which shows he made a later revised edition.

8. Nonetheless, homosexuals condemn themselves until they consider the forces that have induced them to this vice. Nowadays science is inclined to consider homosexuality as a disease, a psycho-physical-biological disorder caused by many factors but above all by a stimulating diet.

9. A known case to consider is the German steamship Neptune that in 1903 lost its propeller and just drifted at sea for a long time. They used up all their living calories found in fresh vegetables, fruits and cereals, so that the crew had to eat dead calories found in boiled preserves, meats, beef jerky, sausages, cold cuts, smoked meat, ham, fish etc. Also they drank all sorts of fine liquors that they were transporting in large quantities in their storerooms like whisky, cognac, port, wine, beer, etc. And

because they were transporting many bales of Bolivian coca leaf most of them chewed it to quench their thirst, still their hunger and forget about this conflictive situation. They also transported a large stash of Havana cigars that they smoked which stimulated them further.

10. This diet was so stimulating that it favored the abnormal development and growth of certain glands which convulsed in the blood of the veins of these rough sailors dragging them into an orgy of homosexuality. Some of them preferred suicide rather than be forced by their companions into such a repugnant vice.

11. The doctor on board in his report said that these men moved around like zombies, dazed, always irritated, puffing like locomotives with excess pressure that escaped in spurts from the security valve.

12. Finally a strong wind pushed the boat to the coast of Panama, where the crew could eat the right foods again and this returned them to health, in other words living calories that are found only in fresh greens, vegetables, fruits and cereals all of which they consumed in large quantities. These living vitamins had the virtue of calming the excitement of these sailors changing them back to normalcy. It was if they were awakened from a lethargic dream state of a horrible nightmare.

14. All of them were completely ashamed what they had participated in during this collective drunken binge, in acts so shameful and repugnant that now in their right minds they sincerely deplored and vehemently condemned. The doctor added that during the rest of their long trip not one sailor backslide into homosexuality.

15. If any cities for their unfavorable geographic location or for any natural or man-made disaster don't have access to foods that have living calories such as fresh greens, vegetables, fruits and cereals and are forced to consume for long periods of time dead vitamins that are found in all types of meats, preserves or in other words all canned food and boiled food, they will find themselves swept away like the sailors on the German boat called Neptune, carried away to such a deplorable vice, such an annihilator of vital force.

16. This is because such unnatural food decomposes the blood, it toxifies it, dirties it, which creates leukemia, which is cancer of the blood, the putrefaction of this precious and vital liquid and it also creates internal putrefaction which manifests in external

putrefaction, in other words a grave moral putrefaction.
17. Nowadays the cities and governments are well informed about the precise causes that lead to this deplorable vice and also about the most effective remedy to fight off this evil in order to save the citizens from complete moral decadence.
18. The principle remedy consists in starting an active education campaign for all citizens including talks on radio programs, articles in newspapers and magazines and the printing of informative brochures. This education campaign must make the people see what a collective disaster this wasteful, destroyer of human energy can cause.
19. At the same time, the governments should concern themselves about how to give the people the precise food that the human body normally needs, advising them that all our lives we can live healthy and strong if we eat nothing more than raw vegetarian food.
20. The principle food of humans is raw vegetarian foods which give the maximum strength to men giving them the vital force, virility and health and not only humans but also the strongest animals that tread the earth such as the bull, the horse, camels, elephants, etc.
21. To eat a vegetable is to eat a piece of the sun, because vegetables absorb the sun's rays which they incorporate within their tissue and this stored energy is given to the people that in turn eat these sun charged vegetables (fruits and grains also come from vegetation) giving them a vigorous vitality.
22. If we plant grains of wheat, beautiful green plants will be produced. But if these grains are boiled first and then planted, nothing will come forth and we will find a rotten seed in the soil.
    This is because life only comes from what is living
          and death comes from that which is dead.
23. To illustrate to the people about these basic truths of life in order to launch an energetic repression of this dangerous vice, will assure the people of a pure and moral life, saving them from the horrendous ordeal that Sodom and Gomorrah suffered.
Chapter 30:
8. Unfermented Grape juice is an excellent natural beverage that strengthens one and doesn't make one drunk like fermented grape juice which has the intoxicant alcohol in it. But the best of all drinks is pure water because this can never be surpassed by any artificial drink made by man.

Also, you must overcome table salt because it's poisonous to the human body, as science has demonstrated. Millions of people and animals too, have never eaten salt and they are in the best of health. They would have died if salt were so indispensable to their health. Nonetheless, the human body needs vegetable salt and not mineral table salt. Mineral salt cannot be assimilated by the body because it lacks the right atomic vibration which only vegetable salt has. Mineral salt when it passes through a living plant, receives an accelerated atomic vibration, transforming it into vegetable salt. Mineral salt is deposited like garbage inside the body especially in the arteries, provoking the dangerous disease called arteriosclerosis, high blood pressure and also blindness, deafness, dementia, etc. Vegetable salt that is found naturally in all vegetables and fruits is easily assimilated by the body, is very healthy, it disintoxicates and purifies the blood, the tissues, lowers and normalizes blood pressure, gives health, vitality and strength, preserves good eyesight, hearing and the mind in a clear, sharp, awakened state to a very advanced age.

+

PARADISIAN NEWSLETTER ++++++ (EDITORIAL NOTES)

THE GREAT MASTER KUKUREPA WHO LIVED ON AN ISLAND

In the history of the Great White Brotherhood, Lodge and Order of Gurus, the most renown of Tibetan Masters, who happened to be of Kagyu lineage, was Marpa. He studied under Naropa, who had been abbot of Nalanda University, the greatest center for Buddhist studies that the world has ever known. Naropa taught Marpa who in turn, was the teacher of Milarepa, Tibet's Great Yogi, Saint and most renown Guru. Thru the most improbable difficulties, Marpa had raised himself from farmer to the status of local clergy, the equivalent of a college professor, doctor or lawyer in the west, and then he made a difficult journey to India. By the time Marpa reached India, Naropa had retired to a simple forest dwelling in Bengal, and altho reputed as one of the greatest of Buddhist Saints, Marpa was disappointed by his humble mean, expecting a more religious setting. But Marpa paid him and explained that he was a priest and farmer in Tibet, not willing to give up this life he chose, and wanted the teaching to translate into Tibetan to make money on it. Naropa agreed easily, gave the instruction, all going very smoothly. When Marpa joined his journey-companion from Tibet to return, comparing teachings acquired, Marpa learned his efforts were worthless. They already had what he had studied in Tibet, but his companion had found a fantastic higher teaching given by the greatest of Gurus. When Marpa told Naropa of this, Naropa explained he could only get that from Kukurepa, who lived in the middle of a lake of poison. Marpa by now was desperate, so he made the journey to the island in the Lake of Poison to such an extraordinary teacher and evidently great mystic to be able to live where he did. But what Marpa found was even more disheartening.

Kukurepa was only an old man who lived in filth midst hundreds of female dogs. The situation was outlandish to say the least, but when Marpa tried to talk to Kukurepa, all he got was gibberish, nonsense. Not only was Kukurepa unintelligible, but Marpa had to be on guard against the hundreds of bitches. Making friends with one, another would growl and threaten him by snapping at him. Marpa, almost beside himself, gave up altogether trying to take notes or getting any secret doctrine. But as soon as Marpa lost hope, Kukurepa began to talk intelligibly in a coherent voice, and the dogs stopped harassing him, and Marpa thus was able to get the extraordinary course.

But when Marpa joined his Tibetan companion, and they started the long trek back, crossing a river, Marpa began telling about how now he had obtained an even more valuable teaching. Becoming jealous, feeling uncomfortable and restless, and complaining about the excess baggage of Marpa's prized manuscripts as he shifted to accommodate himself, he tipped the boat and they lost everything... When Marpa got back to Tibet, he had nothing but many stories to tell of his travels and studies, but nothing solid to prove his knowledge and experience but unbelievable tales. What's more he gradually realized that his written notes only covered parts of the teachings that he had not understood. What he understood, he had had no need of writing down, because it was a part of his own experience and part of him in practice. Realizing this, Marpa lost his desire to gain riches from a teaching, or be a prestigious teacher, now really seeking Enlightenment. He saved up gold till he had enough to again travel to India, but now found Naropa cold and hostile. When Marpa offered him only the major portion of his gold, Naropa asked for all of it, and then given more and more ending up with inferring that Marpa was trying to buy his high teaching by deception.

Once all the bags of gold were given Naropa threw the gold away, tossing it about in the air: "What need have I of gold. The whole world is gold for me!" This was a moment of great opening for Marpa however: he opened up, giving up preconceptions and prejudices and became able to absorb all the great teaching. Not only do you have to be able to give up all of one's material possessions, but all the mistaken concepts one has from the past, to be able to readily absorb the complete Truth when it is given. Mastery is one continual process, of finding openings into the falsely educated mind, prejudice-bound to new learning, and only when we forsake all hope attached to past sensual training, by surrendering completely do we realize that the whole thing was not a lot of gibberish and snapping bitches.

We have briefly retold a 1970 lecture given at Boulder, Colo., U.S.A. therapeutic community by Chogyam Trungpa, former abbot of Surmang Lamasary of Marpa lineage in Tibet. I wish all the disillusioned people who spend funds and efforts to come here hoping I would have time to talk to them or expecting a great University or other marvel, had read stories like the one above. Great Masters appear as ordinary and full of faults as those who are disappointed judging them, expecting something else, or in other words, it takes a Master to recognize a real Master. Moreover, there are many who wish they could study here with me as if that would solve things. Yet, I am a great believer in discipline, or a DISCIPLINARIAN, demanding so much that very few could ever come up to my demands. Studying our courses, and teaching yourself, avoids a bossy disciplinarian. In fact, if you can even support reading my courses, you do better than average, not to speak of the abuse and displeasure practice will cause you. What the Eastern Vajrayana and Dhyan, Ch'an or Zen schools taught about Paradoxes such as "Abide in the Abode of the Non-Abiding", was taught in ancient Greece (535 B.C.) by Heraclius, who said, "That which is at variance with itself, agrees with itself." Life is a Paradox. Good depends on evil, and Truth depends on error, Life is dependent on this process of dying to ourselves, Illumination on overcoming illusions. In Western logic, if anything or everything were rational, Life would lose its purpose, not having anything to teach us or for us to learn. The opposites cancel one another, and Life ceases to manifest,- Nirvana, Illumination or the Void.

When we open up, really surrender to Cosmic Will or LOVE ALL, we are ready to give up past prejudices, publicly confess our sins and foolish errors to help all others on the Path. Selfishness or egotism causes people to cover up their errors, trying to be so artificially consistent. When someone reveals one's secret sins in public especially, it offends or mortally injures one worse than a whiplashing or physical wound. Traditionally, in Western monasteries, the head disciplinarian of a Rule like the Trappists, have had to discipline members actually with a whiplashing which willingly they knew they deserved. Because modern society encourages avoiding pain, using pain-killers, pacific persuasion by rationalization, logical arbitration about Truth, the world keeps compromising till everything ends in confusion and self suicide. In 1945, when I began writing, I warned "Words were constructed to conceal the Truth", and later in Transcendental Truth Teachings, I admitted Truth cannot be told,- simply because it is not consistent or logical. Life is transforming eternally, only change being permanent. My own life story on the physical plane is of the same lot, and some think even more unfortunate, as to other flesh and blood. The fruit of physical pitfalls in the lessons learned, the wisdom gained and Eternal Spiritual Plenitude of Consciousness is the real Worth.

On September 17th 1977, the ad hoc members of The Pristine Order of Paradisian Perfection called together, altho not "to order", a meeting in which they openly declared they did not abide by the Inner Ordinance or Rule of the Order. They frankly now admitted they only wanted legal status, so as to remain in Ecuador as "Paradisian Missionarios" or workers, evading government restrictions against increasing Immigrants, privileges without penalties, as if that solved problems for themselves and those wanting to join them. Those concerned now wanted no restrictions on diet, a free hand in what they were doing, and did not want to be any part of the "Sublimest and Strictest Discipline on earth", which they had joined supporting, to get approval, which now caused them displeasure. The rich being able to enjoy all pleasures seek suicide: Love is not pleasure-seeking. The Gates of Paradise do not open just because you have a few thousand dollars to spend, and you feel cheated if you are not accepted as a member because you cannot live up to the diet and Rule. As Rajneesh wrote in "Hidden Harmony", "Life is not a problem to be solved, but a mystery to be lived." This is the point in the Strictest Discipline. Do you LOVE LIFE, or prefer to enjoy all you desire and crave? Why join a discipline and Order if you cannot honestly tolerate those principles of seeking Illumination of the Founder? Why pretend what you aren't? People are not even able to live up to the Rule outside the Order, and yet they seem to imagine just joining us without freedom, being forced, they will obey the Rule. On the contrary, all I can say is "You are not a Paradisian, so run along back to your cities and food pleasures, but without further pretext as being one of us." Remember that "Whom the Lord loveth, he chasteneth, he scourgeth everyone he receiveth. Persevere under DISCIPLINE.."

My mother deeply loved me, and could not tolerate anyone physically beating me but she had a better way. When I misbehaved, she told visitors about my acts of mischief, and I know how it hurt to have my sins revealed in the background of her acts of loving kindness, so inconsiderate of her selfless love. Is Discipline out of style in the 20th century? One of the axioms of Modern Science is that the Scientific Discipline of any experiment or system proves its worth in practicality. We do not pretend to be Logical, altho Logos is revealed in the Hidden Harmony.

At the time of the September 17th meeting it was a Paradox... at headquarters, much worse than seeking Peace living in a Volcano, claimed of the "Saint of the Andes". I was incarnating Kukurepa living here on my symbolic island in a Lake of Poison, in the "Sacred Valley of Longevity". The neighbors to the south and west had been spraying for nearly a decade, trying an arsenal of agro-chemicals, on demonstration to educate the valley inhabitants and neighbors to the east followed by poisoning my irrigation water by their run-off from sprayed crops which caused severe illness till I had to give up irrigating to avoid the poison, which stunted production. The farmer right at the entrance to our Paradise began spraying former pasture planted to beans. To top that, as I felt my body stiffen from spray drift, another neighbor to the east began creating a breathing problem with diesel (crude) oil fumes by a malfunctioning motor in his raw sugar cane grinding mill. The diesel fumes ended 3 weeks later when he had harvested his crop but was followed by another farmer burning brush to clear land. The only solution to all these problems would be the formerly planned move to

"Shambhala" lands, which after visiting the region, in a recent journal I pondered about another possible "Mirage in the desert". Worse, rather than giving any compassionate support as said to be the purpose of the Sept. 17th meeting, the group was outright hostile, telling me that I should pay back the cost of the land to the donor. This was the Ultimate, I could not go there in peace without upsetting those who once pretended to become disciples under a discipline I founded as the Order. Both Shambhala and New Eden lands were impractical, to me at least, and worse by going there, I became a participant in the money wasting decision, I had been against, and now I was to be punished for a third bad decision in buying land they insisted on buying against my will... To top it, after their glowing description, I had published the same in my journal, and I was blamed for space and support I gave to what I was not able to verify, due to my handicap preventing the long hikes to see the lands.

One of the former members, rather than repenting their diet violations that give Vitalogical chastity, wrote me, "We all have your ideals, but Gods and Goddesses don't need 'The Strictest Discipline on earth'. Discipline is for Sinners. As long as we are building Paradises all over, why not let it stand at that?" To say the least, such a concept of my teaching is COMPLETELY WRONG. Super-market builders in Loja called what they had done "El Paraiso", and many who oppose the Vitalogical Sciences, are also building Paradises by planting nut groves, etc. Gods and Goddesses are the Spiritually REBORN initiates, without menses or seminal losses, living on living food, not from hot soup pots, dead and seminal substances, cheese, and such things. "Whosoever is born a God, committeth not sin because their SEED ABIDETH WITHIN THEM, and they cannot sin because they are born of God. In this the children of God and children of the Devil are distinguished." (I-John 3:9) The whole concept of the Lovewisdom Message sets it apart from all other teachers, and there are hundreds who have failed in Paradise Building colonies of the past. My strict adherence to discipline has the objective of avoiding past errors, rather than repeat them, as our expelled or former members insisted in repeating. None of those former members applied for studies to become Initiates Spiritually, or got their Doctor of Vitalogical Sciences degree as the INNER ORDINANCE or Rule of our Order requires, which requires living by strict dietetic rules and not having sexual losses, writing theses showing complete understanding and mastery of these principles. Unless one is Spiritually gifted, Spiritually Entranced in this work, it is difficult or impossible, so why pretend you are a member of the Heavenly Hierarchy, Gods, etc. The Spiritual or White Brotherhood or Order of Gurus guiding mankind are not just weak-willed folk seeking refuge from civilization, so why join us. If you are capable, you are a PROVEN GURU and are able to live up to the Rule, and detest and abhor living the wrong way so much that our Yoga or "Yoke is sweet and burden light".

The PRISTINE ORDER OF PARADISIAN PERFECION are Gods and Goddesses living at our "Camp of the Saints" in the Strictest Discipline on earth, guiding the Destiny of mankind. Unless one conquers lower appetites, desires, craving in self, it cannot do anything for others, guide them, or Save or Rescue man from his present dilemma.

The SECONDARY ORDER OF THIS PARADISIAN PERFECTION are individuals living the Strictest Discipline alone like hermits in their own Paradisian Retreats.

The TERTIARY ORDER OF THIS PARADISIAN PERFECTION are those who started wrong getting married, raising children, etc. but repent and now live up to our Strictest Discipline. Needless to say, the Pristine Order living under the founder's direction has its Inner Rule and government approved Statutes authorizing the Inner Ordinance, the Vitalogical Sciences, and teachings of the Founder. The sponsors of the Order, students and subscribers to publications are not who determine the Strictest Discipline, and donors and candidates in no way oblige the Order to care for them, but are here on trial. We are not an Asylum for the Homeless and Refugees. We have arranged for the establishment of the LOVEWISDOM FOUNDATION in the U.S.A. where our books and teachings, beside our journal shall be published and distributed in the future. This will involve world-wide publicity, T.V., etc. all of which does not help in ridding the evils of civilization, trying to establish the example. Thus, we must become, as we preach, an ESOTERIC SANCTUARY where only the Elect shall be invited. Possibly in the next few journals you shall be given the address and instructions. Henceforth subscriptions and books will be mailed by the Foundation, and centers which publish our teachings in other nations and languages in Sweden, France,

England, Argentina, Chile, Mexico, Canada, etc. as in the past. We will no longer attend to letters coming here with a note saying, "Please send us all the Free Information you have available". We have data from the past, out-dated and a dollar is not enough postage to mail it. Only students having completed courses of study and who live by our discipline will be invited to the Inner Esoteric Sanctuary, and this present location will be another error we preach against making.

MAHA MAITREYANA MANDALA

"Maha" is Great or High, "Maitreya" refers to the Super-Conscious Illumination or aspects of the New Age Lovewisdom Message of the Avatar, Buddha and Christ, and "Yana" is the Vehicle or School supporting same. "Mandala is the Circle or Center, which altogether connotes "NEW AGE WORLD SPIRITUAL CENTER", since the Great White Brotherhood, Lodge and Order was transferred from Tibet to the High Andes, where we speak of it as the Higher Heavenly Hierarchy.

In 1942, the arrival of the New Age and activities of the Great White Brotherhood in the Andes was published in books from Columbia - Chile in the Andes: (1) "Factores y Beneficios de la Iniciacion Espiritual por El Tibetano, Maestro K.H. Pr. O.M. Chenrezi Lind (Bogota) (2) "Plan Evolutivo del Mundo", por Samariter, Orden Samaritana Internacional, Casilla 1763, Santiago de Chile. "Samariter" is the pen-name of Martin Slotosch Loth, who brought the Samaritan Order to the Andes of Chile from Germany and seems to be who translated "El Evangelio de la Salud de San Juan" (Healing God Spell of Saint John) into Spanish, just as Emil Mogner has been accused of the German translation made in 1899 from the Aramaic Original, since the Order officially holds these matters confidential. (3) The American Weekly published the version of Lamas, etc. in the Andes, the Father of the New Race and Age, etc. 1942 to 1944, but distorted. In the Spiritual Initiation of Lovewisdom, in the "Maitreya" book you may have wondered about the prophetic symbol of the PUMA, the Mountain Lion of the High Andes, known also as the Panther or cougar in the U.S., being a lion without the mane of the species living in Asia and Africa. Leo, or Lion is the Lovewisdom initiatic symbol as well as that of the Living Buddha (Kut Humi LAL SINGH), the above sketch giving a view of our Esoteric Sanctuary terrain, a lion of Asia (with mane like (J.L.) with a Paradisian companion approaching in the background, but pumas and poisonous serpents are whom we choose to live with. You may have heard about recent nuclear bomb tests at Lop Nor and former Eastern Esoteric Sanctuary sites of the White Brotherhood, Lodge and Order, but now in the High Andes our Esoteric site is within the 50 kilometer border area north from Peru where only Ecuadorian citizens can reside. This will avoid Yanquis with their dollar and "free" concepts moving in on us. In no way can people pretend to join, until they are familiar with life in Ecuador, beside becoming initiated in the Vitalogical Sciences by thesis and experiences living in the Strictest Discipline.

The higher reaches of the river valley contain hidden hollows 2,000 to 2,500 m. of sites unseen by man due to rugged terrain of jagged peaks reaching 3,000 meters at most, being ideal for orchards of groups of trees of subtropic and temperate warm regions, dry and windy. Then there is an abrupt drop of the river stream over falls levelling out to 1,500 meters (lower than our place at Sukhavata) with dry, sunny climate that takes away gloom and shadows of cloudy or humid opposites. The soil is sandy and stony insuring mineral richness and aeration of the roots that fruit trees prefer. Former inhabitants left silent reminders of rock wall fences still intact, avocado trees that yielded 10,000 per crop whose giant trees we will be partaking of, beside cherimoyas, guavas, rose apples, oranges, limes, lugma sapotes and other goodies turning up with each exploration by a faithful Scribe of our Order. Buddha received Enlightenment sitting under a "ficus religiosa" or Bodhi Tree and the climate is ideal for figs, beside grapes and dry Calif. climate fruits. Plans are being drafted for a Scriptorium or Library for thousands of rare books we have collected for the Archives, where the Masters of Wisdom may concur, study, write and prepare manuscripts to be distributed to centers publishing our works around the globe for guidance of mankind in the New Age. Basically, the location answers our needs of Sanctuary, without attending to novices who complain about the Strictest Discipline, having the needed atmosphere for Spiritual Entrancement for Disciples who find Godly goals and Supreme Joy living the Perfect Way.

"SHAMBHALA"

"First will begin an unprecedented war of all nations (World War I, II). Afterwards brother shall rise against brother, oceans of blood shall flow (as witnessed in present civil terrorism). Only a few years shall lapse before everyone shall hear the mighty stamps of the Lord of the New Era, Maitreya. The Banner of Shamballa (Camp of the Saints) shall encircle the Central Lands (Ecuador) of the Blessed One," wrote Guru Avananda. Mdme. Blavatsky added that after North America is destroyed by earthquakes and "volcanic" (nuclear blast) fire, the New Race, the 7th Race will appear on the 7th Continent, South America, characterized by a complete clairvoyant development.

"In the Era of Maitreya, the World Teacher,- Now,- flowers shall bloom in profusion and out of season and women shall wear them. Music and dance of South America shall become predominant. The country named Ecuador S.A. will become the SPIRITUAL CENTER, the Tibet of the West, after Maitreya the World Teacher has established himself over all the Earth under the Banner of Maitreya,- which is Truth and Justice for all Earthlings. OM MANI PADME HUM." The Red Lama (Sungma Oracle) copyrighted this in his ETERNAL FOUNTAIN in 1947, while I was in my Temple of Metta-Aum Initiation, at Lake Quilotoa, having been guided to it by a vision of a natural temple of a lake within a mountain peak with the Ogdoad Symbol: which the Red Lama commented saying "The Cathedral of Nature is the True Church for man, and the human body is the Temple of Divine Universal Spirit." The Founder of Theosophy, Mdme. Blavatsky, described SHAMBHALA as a mysterious place due to Prophetic Events. It is mentioned in the Puranas as where the Kalki Avatar will appear. The Kalki Avatar is the last of Manvantaric incarnations of Vishnu. He is the MAITREYA Buddha of Buddhists and Soshish, the Savior of the Zoroastrian Parsis, but of whatever religion, he returns on a white horse, etc. is the Word of God, the HEALER (Jesus) of Nations comes calling all those cleansed with blood-juice of Paradisian fruits (Vitalogy!)

In his Wesak Message of 1942, Master Kut Humi Lal Singh, Prince O.M. Cherenzi Lind, the Tashi Lama which H.P.B. (Mdme. Blavatsky) credits as the Head of the GREAT WHITE BROTHERHOOD, since he created the office of Daila Lama who attends to outer political affairs,-- announced the beginning of the New Aquarian Age, the Spiritual (Bodha) Renaissance, and coinciding with my Day of Spiritual Birth, Dec. 13th, 1942. So together with the Sungma Red Lama, they jointly declared unity in Spirit behind the Advent and Banner of Lovewisdom, the Western translation of Maitreya Buddha. It should be explained that Kut Humi is the Master of the Hyperborean Race (name historically given to the Finnic Race) in relation to the 2nd Ray, which is that of LOVE-WISDOM, according to Archives of old H.P.B. quotes. Also, K.H. personal stationary (in our archives) gives the Flag or Banner of Love-Wisdom, as that of the Spiritual Grand Lodge and Eternal Orient (meaning of Great White Brotherhood), with an embossed seal showing his identity as "Tashi Hutulktu Kwang Hsih" and signature of Prince O.M. Cherenzi Lind in America and "Schernrezig-Lind in Europe,- Tibetan being impossible to translate. Tashi Hutulktu is the Tashi Lama, while "CHENREZI", said to be the Celestial Son of Amitabaha which both refer to incarnations of the Logos, equivalent of the Patriarch Archbishop, Pope, etc. being the Head Vicarage of Christ Incarnate in Christian terms of the West. Combined Eastern Christians and Buddhists established the Lama Hierarchy of the Great White Brotherhood. "KWAN HSIH" of the Tashi Lama refers to the Prince of Ch'an office, head of the Largest Buddhist Denomination, located at Ch'An Cheng Lob, Tiwa, Sin-Kiang, Northern Tibet, and is the Chinese Buddhist term for logos Incarnate in Male Principle. Kwan Yin is the Logos Incarnate in female principle, which Anagarika Nirgidma King, used in her published works as President of the Bodha Society of America Inc., or Violet Blossom Reed who "mothered" me in the Maitreyana Initiations. Thus, the Kwan Shi Yin and Kwan Yin, are given the equivalent of "CHRISTOS-SOPHIA" in Christian Gnostic terminology by H.P.B., explaining to our readers how it relates to our group. Both the letters of Pr. Chenrezi and Violet Blossom refer to myself as their Spiritual Son and their Dear Disciple as well as Cosmic Brother, which accounts for so much criticism my early writings offer my Teachers because of the Inner Wisdom nature, and not knowing the meaning of titles and names given to the High Initiations I received living as a Hermit, oblivious to the prophetic mission they prepared for the Lovewisdom Message spiritually. Their guidance was preceded by the Universal Spiritual Union and the Great Universal Spiritual Brotherhood (Maha Bodha Mandala) started in 1913 that began the largest Buddhist Movement in history, claiming 800 million. (When training as Maitreya)

EPILOGUE

"Only Living Food Gives Life and Joy of Living!" "The God-Endowed" (The 1976 version had a drawing of John with eleven stars around his head, with the above captions.)

"The Healing God Spell of St. John" of the Samaritans, Gnostics or Primitive Christians of St. John, originating in the Essene Order of Mt. Carmel, had been intended for the Healing of the physical body, but there was more, a Spiritual or Metaphysical Healing Scripture and doctrine also, in the teachings of the illumined John. Combining The Healing God Spell with the "GOLDEN TEXT OF THE HOLY GRAIL", presented in the book "NEW LIGHT IN AN OLD LANTERN", gives one an all-sided view of Salvation in the New Spiritual Age thru Regeneration. Today's Holy Bible hardly does any of that: The first chapters tell about the Pristine order of Paradisian Perfection as a foundation, but from there on, with the descent of the human race into sin, the Scriptures become confused, and the Truth lumbers under the burden of ignorance. We have sought to dedicate much of this work to purging and removing the undesired physical weight gained by ignorance, and likewise the mental problems concerning the Scriptures and their authors, but now we would like to give a foretaste of Spiritual Insight into Illumination in the teachings of John.

"THE GOLDEN TEXT OF THE HOLY GRAIL" or "THE PRIMITIVE GOSPEL RESTORED"
as rendered by Joseph C. Bonner (1900-1963)

John 1: The Principle is Activity in your Immortal Spirit. The Active Principle is adnate to the Deity, which is the One Eternal Principle. It is the First Emanation of the God-head. All things are manifest by IT, and not one thing exists without IT. IT is the LIFE and the LIGHT of all Mankind. Altho this Immortal Light is aglow within the Unenlightened yet they fail to realize it. There appeared a Celestial Being, an Emanation of Deity, called the God-Endowed (Yohanan, John). This one made himself manifest to testify to the existence of Immortality in order that others, by his act, might know. He was not the Active Principle, but appeared only to bear witness of emanating Embodied Light. This is the True Light which, when united with a mortal, enlightens that sentient being. It is already within our "little world" (microcosmos) for thru IT the individual evolves, while the "worldly" know not why. IT is bound up in the "I", yet the individual fails to realize "I" from "IT", but to those who do, IT gives to them the Power TO BE; "Reborn" as children of Deity, those who know they are--something more than just a person physically, born of carnal desire by the will of man, -- a Divine Being. When the Divinity becomes activated within us, we can behold IT'S Radiation, emanating from incarnate beings who have become "reborn",- One with the Father,- consumed with the Oneness of Reality. Because of its universality all can partake of this "Eternal Gift", instead of "Temporal Gifts". Natural Law is taught by every Liberated One, but Godliness, in fact is attained only thru Union with "+" (the Immortal Divine Spirit), your Illuminator. No one can see Deity, the Un-manifest, ever! Only the Shining One, the First Emanation of the God-head, is revealed. Such is the testimony of THE GOD-ENDOWED, John.

+++

Brother Bonner further comments: "The God-Endowed (Yohanan) broke thru the veil of illusion and became conscious of the Divine World as any mortal in any age can. He repudiated the false teachings that it is gained in some after life when one loses his outer vesture. No Messiah, or Maitreya, will ever free mankind. (Luke 22:45) Yeshu went up the mountain (of consciousness) and meditated deeply until he obtained Union with Divinity, the Spiritual part of soul (nous), freeing him from Naphesh, the animal or desire part of the soul." Christ is the name of "+".

CHAPTER I Prantara-Ghoshanam THE CRY IN THE WILDERNESS

While helplessly meandering about this spiritless wilderness, the WORD of Deity manifest itself to one who became God-Endowed, making him a son of the "Father of Waters". After that the God-Endowed came out of the wilderness and went along the shores of the Jordan proclaiming his Lustration and Reformation, misconceptions having been wiped away, and all his doctrine was: "Change your view". The Divine Theocracy is here, -- Now! People came from the surrounding countryside, even the Sacred City, to hear him reveal "the Well" in their midst that turns one away from all wrong action into the Way of Peace. The God-Endowed wore the cherished garb of a Patriarch, cloaked about his hairy body with (a hemp rope) apron fastened about his waist, and his food was what this wilderness yielded. As the people were taught to await a Divine Incarnation, they wondered about this God-Endowed (John), whether or not he was the "Expected" (Messiah, Meshaykah in Aramaic; Maitreya in Sanskrit). Ultimately the Ecclesiastical Court, hearing of this Seer-Evangelist, sent their priests and elders from the Sacred City to interrogate him. When he observed those Tsadukim (Sadducees) ritualists decrying him for teaching the Divine Lustration, "You cult of Serpent - charmers!" he cried, "Who forewarned you to flee from the retributive force of your Karmic acts? The Reapers scythe even now is striking at the root of your 'Trees', like any other tree that does not bring forth its fruit is cut down for firewood. You had better mature that spiritual fruit, which gives one the right to wear religious garb and expect no immunity by supposing that A - BRAHAM will Father you, for let me tell you that the 'ALL-Father' is able to raise up from these Arabians, sons with a holiness greater than yours!" "Who are you", they retorted, "The Expected?" Emphatically he denied it, "I am NOT!" "Then who are you, - Elijah?" "No!" he replied. "Then who are you?" they insisted, "Give us an answer that we can deliver to those who sent us. Whom do you consider yourself to be?" "Tell them," he replied, "I AM THAT,-- which is written in the book of Spiritual Vision (Isaiah): "A Voice calling from out of the Silence: prepare to meet thy Beloved! Be found worthy of that Exultant Life. Raise up that which is in the low place! Draw down that which is on high. Then your obstacle is removed and the hard sought goal is won. Let everyone unite with their 'Beloved'! Bring forth the Shining One for all mankind to see thy Immortal Spirit made manifest!" Those sent to interrogate him said, "If you are neither the 'Expected', nor a God-Incarnate (Elijah) nor that Foreteller, why do you perform the Sprinkling Rite?" The God-Endowed replied, "I lustrate them to the Great Waters about them for a 'Change of Mind' then, following this, there comes a mightier consciousness far superior, which even I have not become like-minded enough to grasp the many ways of his Wisdom. It is He who will lustrate you with the sacred fire from the holy fire of the Holy Spirit. This Fan-Bearer winnows the chaff from the wheat to gather the kernel On High while the husks are consumed by His Fire." The Commoners that had gathered were now astir asking, "What shall we do?" "You have 'two coverings', he replied, "unburden yourself of one! And, whoever has Spiritual Bread, share it with others! The men of

Learning and the orthodox religionists officially occupy the Chair of the Law-giver (Moses). Therefore, give heed and practice whatever precepts they tell you, but do not match your conduct with their actions for they only preach what they practice. Besides, they think up heavy unportable burdens for you to shoulder which they could not so much as stagger about with, themselves. They only flaunt gaudy amulets and add extra tassels to their robes. All their religious performances are only to create a spectacular effect. They insist on being seated at the head couch at festive meals and the highest ranking seats at the Assemblies. To be made obeisance to publicly in the market place and addressed as "RAV" (Teacher). Never call them Rav for only the EXPECTED (Messiah) is your teacher, and call no earthly man "Father", for you have only one who dwells on High and all of you are His children. Let me tell you, unless your Virtue greatly exceeds that of the learned and the religionists, you will never attain to the Realm of the Divine." Others sought his Lustrations but being merchants, asked, "What must we do?" "Charge no more than what is just," he replied, "And do not accumulate earthly treasure for yourselves, which moths and corrosion destroy, or for thieves to steal. Sell your surplus without regret and provide yourselves with the purse that never wears out. Possess the Heavenly Treasure that is endless where no thief can venture and no moth can ruin, for whatever treasure you have, your consciousness will be dwelling upon it.

Be not anxious about Life, what you will eat and what you will clothe yourself with. Is not Life more important than food, or the body more than raiment? Look in the air at the feathered birds. They neither sow nor reap nor store up food because your Father on High feeds them. Are you not more superior than birds? Tell me, which of you by holding a thought can add one cubit to your stature? If you have not even power to do that, why be anxious about other matters. Consider how the desert lilies grow, they neither weave nor spin. Yet I say to you not even "Solomon" clothed with all His Radiance is to be compared with these. Therefore, if The Unspeakable can clothe the fields with herbage one day, only to be used to fire the bake-oven tomorrow, will he not clothe you much more? You faithless! So stop being concerned about "What should I eat", or "What should I wear". That is all that worldly people are interested in. The KNOWER on High knows what you need. Therefore just seek the Divine

155 The Healing God Spell of Saint John

Realm, and everything will come to you. So stop taking thought about tomorrow for it will bring its own anxieties. Each day brings its own trouble.

Those called to duty as soldiers asked, "What are we to do?". "The virtue of a law-enforcement officer is to be manly, therefore, do not spy or falsely accuse others with threats or violence to extort, but be content with your pay." He continued to address the postulants with many other admonitions. All this occurred at the place of affiliation (Bethany) beside the Jordan where the God-Endowed was lustrating. (The Aramaic word for baptizing means lustrating, since the Initiator 'Baptist' did not dip with water, but his disciples did, which shows how words of double meaning were used to create N.T. Bible allegories.)

CHAPTER II Aisvara - Sanskaras THE DIVINE INAUGURATION

He went out from there, accompanied by his companions, and came to his native village where he had been reared. On the Rest Day he entered the Temple of the Nazoreans, and, as it is the custom, went up to the reading stand whereupon the God-Freed was handed the Scroll of Spiritual Vision (Isaiah) unrolled at the place for that day's reading.

He began: "The Breath of The Unspeakable is upon me. Because of this I AM ANOINTED and now commissioned: To Herald the Message of The Divine to those who have it not; To arouse their slumbering spirit; To reveal the Way of Emancipation to the enmeshed soul by restoring sight to the Spiritual Eye! To Liberate one from the adverse nature and to proclaim that the appointed time to BE,- is NOW!" Then furling the Scroll, handed it back to the attendant, and, as he returned to his seat every eye in the Temple stared at him for he said: "Today's Scripture reading which you have just heard,- has come to pass in me!"

CONTINUED EPILOGUE

The custodians of the "Healing God Spell of Saint John" have said that in the New Age, this text will complement the Study of the Holy Bible. However, not only do we need the help of the "Healing God Spell" but the Holy Bible itself contains so many changes and additions that to be able to read and understand it ~imitive Christians of the first three centuries did, many
·~ns must be clarified.
le is composed of the "Old Covenant"
the "New Covenant" which is really Covenant

Anew, or "Ancient Restored Teachings". Basically, both the "Covenants" refer to the "BIBLE OF THE WISE MEN FROM THE EAST" (or India), referred to as the "NIVIHIM" or "The Prophets", which were not mere Seers, but rather "Spiritually Illumined" since they were Buddhist Yogis. They dared to teach openly the true or "orthodox" doctrine of Spiritual Illumination meaning Buddhahood. "The members of this school vigorously repudiated the emptiness of blind formulisms and the gory ritualisms performed upon altars in Temples. They preached that the useless slaughter of lambs, doves and other animals was a vain sacrifice. This school, which Jesus (God-Freed) typifies when he denounced the Rabins and their Levites (Priests) for making great emphasis of trivial things, such as the washing of hands, fasting and ceremonial acts, for maintaining commerce even on the very steps of the temples selling doves, incense, candles, lucky tokens and other religious merchandise,- while misleading the people by withholding the real spiritual meanings of the Doctrine," as quoted from "NEW LIGHT IN AN OLD LANTERN" by Joseph Bonner.

This "Bible of the Wise Men", the Initiated or Illumined is the Gnostic Spiritual Doctrine of the WHITE BROTHERHOOD, Lodge (Ekklesia or Church), and most fully revealed in the Essene Order and Colleges of Mt. Carmel, which used the text "Initiation of Ioanaes" (John), meaning of Apocalypse, which is not open to public circulation, like the rest of the Peshitta Aramaic Bible. These were the White Friar Carmelites, known in the O.T. as the "Sons of the Prophets" or NIVIHIM who received the White Mantle of Elias (Elijah) apostolically thru Initiations of Initiates. The Illumined Gnostic Mani, not only established the Doctrine thru-out Persia, but went with the earliest recorded missionaries to Northern Tibet (Turfan Turkistan) establishing Esoteric Doctrine in 272 A.D., enabling the largest Center of Mahayana Buddhism, or Ch'An to later get dominion in the 8th century, or the White Lotus Order of Gurus, etc.

The books of the Holy Bible were given strange untranslated names, which told their significance, but eventually these names were no longer associated with Spiritual Initiations or Teachings, and supposed to be naming NON-EXISTING PROPHETS or their Scriptures. Here is their meaning: FIRST BIBLE (Book of God) consisted of:

(1) GENESIS, The Origin or Principle; (2) EXODUS, The Way

out or The Name: (3) LEVITICUS, Priests or God Spoke; (4) NUMBERS, A District or In The Desert; (5) DEUTERONOMY, The Second Law or The Word (s). This is the TORAH, or The 5 Books of the Law or Doctrine, or orthodox Israelites.

THE MEGILLOTH means Rolls, referring to Legends, read at festivals: (1) Song of Solomon, or Bride and Bridegroom of New Testament; (2) RUTH, or Spiritual Love, human seeking the Divine; (3) LAMENTATIONS, The Mourning of burning of the Temple and City of Jerusalem 50 B.C.; (4) ECCLESIASTES, Preacher, or Oration read at the feast of Tabernacles; (5) ESTHER (Astar) Name of a star, Venus and Myrtle, relating to the Persian era. Purim feast.

THE BIBLE OF THE WISE MEN, Nivihim or Prophets, SECOND BOOK....UNFOLDMENT:

(1) JOSHUA, Iesus (Jesus) or God Freed (Savior); (2) JUDGES, Deliverers, Book of Guides of Mankind, High Bishops; (3) SAMUEL I-II, or Books of the Heavenly Kingdom of God, and Kingdom of Judgement, which are completed with the Kingdom of the Beloved, and the Kingdom of Peace, called (4) KINGS I - , giving FOUR SPIRITUAL KINGDOMS (or Realms.) (5) ISAIAH, Book of Spiritual Vision (not the name of any Prophet), (6) JEREMIA, The God Exalted or only "Book of Prophecy" in the Bible; (7) EZEKIEL, Revelation or Unfoldment; (8) MINOR PROPHETS: Hosea (Help of God), Joel (Almighty) Amos (Pack Carrier), Obadiah (God's Laborer), Jonah (God's Spirit), Micah (Who is like God), Hahum (Comforter), Habakkuk (Love's Embrace), Zephaniah (Mystery of God), Haggai (Festival), Zachariah (Remembered of God), Malachi (God's Divine), which completes the BOOK OF INITIATED.

THIRD BOOK OF BIBLE or "Ketuvim", Non-Canonical Other Writings:

(1) Psalms (Hymns of Praises), (2) Proverbs (Maxims of the Peaceful. HEBREW APOCRYPHA: (1) JOB (The Accuser), (2) DANIEL (Judge me, God), (3) EZRA-NEHEMIA (Divine Help) (4) CHRONICLES (Diaries). This finishes the ancient traditions, handed down thru Egypt and the Far East, telling of a Race of God-men, coming from the Paradise of the Wise Men, but later due to long winters the Patri-archos (Great Fathers) Nivihim, Initiated Gnostics, Essenes, Yogis, Lamas, Magi, etc. went underground (Esoteric). The sons of the rulers of Palestine went to Essene Schools, with John as was the case with Herod Antipas,

who secretly saved John-Jesus from death by beheading and crucifixion, substituting others, to appease the anger of the Jews.

"AUTOBIOGRAPHICAL COMPENDIUM OF ST. JOHN"

Testimony of my Life, incarnate as St. John, if the reader may pardon my intimate feeling of oneness, was made by Flavius Josephus in the year 53 A.D. when he became a disciple of Banus. Banim means sons, and in the aforementioned "Golden Text" (p. 95), where it says "Sons (banim) with holiness greater than yours" (translated incorrectly as "stones" in both Luke and Matt. 3:8-9), it refers to the All-Father as A-Brahm, of which are the Ayran and Jewish people. Along with Philo of Alexandria who held that Essenes, Pythagoreans, Magi, Therapeuts, etc. were missionary brethren with "Gymnosophists" from N.E. India (Buddhist Yogis or "naked philosophers"), the Ayrans, Egyptians and Jews, all derive their legendary origin from Central Northeast Asia, born of God,- Brahman, altho the Lord was considered too Sacred for mortals to name. Josephus invented the term "Jesus Christ", as a Greek equivalent to Aramaic allegories, and "Banus" is evidently a Greek accommodation for "Sons of God" or FIRST CHRISTIANS OF ST. JOHN. The "Sons of the Resurrection" or "Sons of God" (Lk. 20:36), who neither marry nor father children, or Eunuchs, is the identical definition Yogis use for Initiate disciples, "Brahma-charins", of which John was the Illumined (Buddha) Messiah (Maitreya), and his Gnostic Christians learned to turn the Jordan (Ganges) back to the source on the Holy Mount "Hermon" (Himalaya), and many other allegorical legends,- used to tell of Kundalini Serpent Power, Chakras, reincarnation, karma, and other Yoga teachings on the (+) Cross, Yoke or Union with Immortal God.

Irenaeus held that "Jesus" was not "crucified" or dead, living to an advanced age as John, as does the N.T., Koran, Gnostic Scriptures universally, just as in the N.T. he was accused of being the Resurrection of John, altho his disciples knew he was Anointed Savior with Illumination. The Council of Nicea of 325 established the doctrine that it was not Christian to say Jesus was a mortal, died or was born, but an Immortal Son of God forever, even if Josephus claimed he had lived with the same for 3 years in the wilderness, "The Letter killeth, only Spirit maketh live".

"The Golden Text", originated in Hamadan, capital city of Media, India, held in veneration as the "Code of the Initiated", which was brought from Malabar to Antioch, Edessa, etc. and to Essene Colleges, and translated from Sanskrit into Syriac (Western Aramaic), the origin of our translations. I am able to affirm all these things in this life, and so prove my identity with John, tracing the Spiritual Initiation in Illumination (Sambodhi, Buddhahood) on the Jordan at Bethany to Yoga origins. Syria had the earliest branch church at Urfa (Edessa), so that from 45 A.D. to 272, Christianity had its "First Christian State" or government of Christian Gnostic teachings, long before the Church was organized by Rome's Emperors. The falsehood of Simon "Peter" being the Rock or Cornerstone of the Christian Faith, is told by I-Peter 2:7 writing from Babylon, refuting Papal claims Peter went to Rome, just as Savior (John's) rejection of Peter, as Satan, and rejected cornerstone (Matt. 16:23, 21:42). Peter was afraid to go to the Crucifixion, meaning Exaltation in Aramaic, and was unable to give up body-consciousness (Simon, clay pot, not leper, condition or consciousness). True Stone "A-banim" is a play of words with "banim", Sons of God, which the Roman Vulgate N.T. ignores. Only a purified diet of Living Water will explain why the Savior defended Mary who sat with him under the fig tree in the Garden, at Bethany (house of Figs) when Martha scolded her for not serving guests of their brother Simon,- in cooked clay consciousness, needing baked bread, rather than living bread (grapes, figs, etc.) which at the Lord's Supper, the Savior said was his body and blood. The Roman Church accepted by Emperors, sought every way possible to pervert the whole story of the Illumined (Baptist - Buddha) sitting under the Bodhi (ficus religiosa, fig) tree of good fruit that blossomed in Palestine's wilderness with the Messiah (Maitreya's) Message, encouraging non-violence, so they hid the word meanings with town names, personal names and sacred words of censored interpretation and only gave the gory details of the unjust crucifixion, rendering it into a mystery of living after dying on the cross fulfilling Jewish doctrines of Salvation by "the blood of the lamb of God", symbolic of giving one's life to save others. With such a message the New Testament became a tool for shaping young men's minds into becoming willing loyal soldiers for the Holy Roman Empire of the Papacy, later used by every Christian military power, even to fight one another, or save pagan nations (like U.S. military gospel against draft-dodgers, C.O.s and AWOLS). Unwittingly by hiding all the Aramaic allegories and word plays, as well as many that remained in Greek versions even, Jerome's Latin Vulgate thus favored the vulgar soldiering instinct of bestial men, with pagan mysteries of drinking the blood of Salvation in wine, battlefield strategy of the Hindu Gita story of Krishna in the Aryan invasion of India and Jewish invasion of Palestine as a "Promised Land". Unless we understand that the Gymnosophists were Buddhist yogis, and the White Brotherhood, Lodge (Ekklesia) and Order of Gurus in Tibet and Himalayas, had the same origins as the Essenes, Therapeuts, Pythagoreans and Magi, one can always be led astray by doctrines against the GNOSTIC FIRST CHRISTIANS OF ST. JOHN, since both the Gita of Yogis like the Bible of Christians embody vulgar teachings glorifying bloodshed, unlike the pure doctrine of the Buddha which spread thru-out the world without bloodshed.

    The Old Syriac text of the Ancient or Primitive Gospel Restored is a translation of the original single Gospel in Sanskrit, "KRISTNASANGITA" coming from Asiatic Christians of India who took up the Yoke, Yoga or the Cross (+), which is the Greek letter (X) or "Christ" (christcross). The four gospels that followed this Single Gospel introduced the Palestine scene and John, the Illumined Savior, eventually running riot with all kinds of name meanings left untranslated giving contradictions and all manner of miracles, which would embarrass sincere seekers of truth, so to prevent anyone from finding out, Roman Rulers destroyed all the contrary evidence and censored what they could not hide. This early text was used by earliest Mono-phytes, Jacobites, Marcionites, etc. who denied the Savior was God made man, named Jesus, of a human genealogy, instead holding that man makes himself acceptable to God, as John preached on the Jordan, and James, Bishop of Jerusalem. James is the English adaptation for Jacob, and Jacobite Mono-phytes, still teaching from their Peshitta Syriac N.T. Bible, at Antioch, (from whom the official charter of the Apostolic Gnostic Christians gains verification), hold fast to the doctrine that Jesus Christ, God the Father and the Holy Spirit are all One Spirit, Light, or Essence, not three, or a Trinity of Persons.

    James of Jerusalem, in his Protevangelion stated Zachary knew Mary when the Savior was conceived, but when Mary went to live with Joseph, James and his brothers became the brothers of the Savior, just as the Apostles James and John were sons of

God, the Bestower (Zebedee). The story of the Crucifixion was of Simon Peter's Gospel, giving the main part of the First complete Gospel, along with parts from other Gospels and Epistles, which the Essene missionaries of Buddhist-Yoga assembled to form the essential doctrine of Kristna and Buddha combined, realized in John.

Tatian of Samosata, born in the year 110, a disciple of Justin, lived an ascetic life establishing the doctrine of Encrates or "Sons of Resurrection" (Brahmachayra) and abstained from animal flesh. He is usually accused of being the author of the "Diatessaron", the Single Gospel, by the Roman Church, saying he "combined the four into one simple text", and just like the Single Gospel's origin being in India essentially, the Yoga-Buddhist tenets adapted to Palestine scenes with John and his apostles, soon incorporated it as local history forgetting the eastern source. Now, the missions at Malabar, India are regarded as branches of Antioch as the "source", but the Hindus know better. Harnack well established the facts that in Tatian's time there was no N.T. Canon, nor were texts regarded as inspired, and that about 160, the Peshitta, the Greek text and Vetus Italica (old Latin) had appeared.

The first of the Single Gospels to be translated from Syriac (Aramaic) into Greek was done by Marc John (Marcion), along with 10 of Paul's Epistles. As a consequence, Marcion's Primitive Chrestians were found thru-out the whole world, Epiphanius, and Jerome and Augustine regarded him as being a "Man of Letters", a bishop's son. He said it was Paul's Gospel obtained with the approval of James in Jerusalem, who with John's teaching, was the source. Later, Basilides, an Old Testament scholar, used his knowledge representing the "Oracles of Matthias (or Matthews) combining Gnostic allegories with Hebrew prophecies and legend. Valentinus elaborated the most Roman Catholic presentation of the Gnosis, involving Egyptian mysteries, adding the mystical Virgin Mary who gave birth without knowing man.

It was Bardesanes (155-233) of the Valentine school, who was brought up by the Abgars, Kings of Edessa who established the first Christian State, mentioned above, acknowledging the Gnostic Christians of St. John as the true Establisher of Christianity, that published the Codex Nass-aryan more widely.

He studied in early Mahayana Buddhist Universities in India, taught Natural Living basically, beside doctrines of Spiritual Rebirth, Reincarnation, Karma, etc. He wrote "The Hymn of the Robe of Glory", about his quest for Immortal Divine Wisdom (+) whose source is the East. Like Buddha and John, he was educated by Essenes with princes.

Mani (216-275) was brought up by parents who were early followers of the Gnostic Christians of St. John, is the establisher of the FIRST UNIVERSAL (Catholic) CHURCH, and not only a Zoroastrian scholar, but studied in Buddhist Universities in India at the sources of Christian Gnostic doctrines. "In the years of Ardashir King of Persia, I grew up and reached maturity. The Living Paraclete came down to me and spoke to me. In the House of God there is nothing evil." He taught "The Father of Greatness called forth the Mother of Life, and the Mother of Life called forth Primal Man. Primal Man armed himself with five gods or angels, angels of Sunlight, Breath of Life, Water, Fire and Air. This Primal Man went forth from Paradise into the battlefield of the world, to preserve the Peace of the Realm of Light." He then tells how the Avatars were sent out in different ages of Man, "into India thru the apostle Buddha, into Persia thru the apostle Zoroaster, into the land of the west thru the apostle of Jesus (Savior)". He was against marriage to give birth to children. One must not commit suicide, build houses, destroy plants or animal life in Nature except vegetables used for food. Mani is derived from Primal Man, Emanation of the Highest Godhead, the Christ, Buddha, Ormuzd. His teaching established his teaching thru-out Persia, to India, to Turkestan (manuscripts found at Turfan, Northern Tibet, Sin Kiang), to Egyptian schools, Rome and St. Augustine once was a disciple even.

We have also illustrated how jealous pretenders became disciples of the Illumined, hungering for truth, only to later seek personal glory, perverting the original teaching so radically that emperors and even modern rulers could wage wars and commit all nature of sins in the old name of religion. We hope the person who reads these Scriptures may find the True Immortal Divine Spirit within, yet invisible to the human eye, except in Creative Works of love and Wisdom. Likewise, I know from thousands of hours, days and decades of study of all great Esoteric Scriptures and Holy Books, the beautiful meditations and contemplations of Immortal Divine Spirit blossom in a fragrance that gives Delight and Happiness forever. The Messiah or Expected One, is Maitreya now blossoming within the Heart of many of my disciples. In the West and East the Sign or Mark of John is the Greek letter Christ, also meaning Anointed or Messiah of Holy Spirit, which is universally a CROSS, (+), The Sweet and Light Yoke of Yoga, ever reminding one in the simplest way of IMMORTAL DIVINE SPIRIT that it stands for. THE HEALING GOD SPELL OF THE GOD-ENDOWED means Spiritual Entrancement or UNFOLDMENT, the Peshitta description of "Gospel", because it enables one to unfold like the petals of a ROSE REVEALING THE WISDOM emanating the fragrance of LOVE, The Tree Of Life (+) bearing spherical fruits of Living Water...

The Oldest Gospel in existence (Library of Congress, dated 128 A.D.) of Marcion, or Mark (Marc-John) even in the later N.T. version censored by Rome, reads: "There went out to him (John) ALL THE COUNTRY OF JUDEA and all they of Jerusalem and were baptized (illumined) by him on the Jordan, confessing their sins," showing that John was the leading religious Teacher of his time. Then, "After John was taken up, Jesus came into Galilee preaching the gospel of the Kingdom of God and saying "the Kingdom of God is at hand, do penance and believe in the Gospel." From this we see that as John had predicted, after his Spiritual Illumination on the Jordan, the Holy Spirit of God would become fully manifest in his life, as John gave himself completely to God, so the Savior (or "Jesus") could completely manifest in him, BORN AGAIN and ANOINTED (or "Christ") of the Holy Spirit (The Comforter, Gnosis in Greek and being Manaen in Aramaic). The Roman Church Fathers selected only the corrupted versions, suspicious of Essenes originating in the Orient, causing emphasis of "Massacre of Innocents", when people were searched to locate John, escorting him to study with children of the rulers, thus becoming "foster brother of Herod, the tetrarch," at the Essene College of Mt. Carmel;- Similarly, the beheading and crucifixion stories were created in common gossip of profane public, conditioned by the bloody sacrifices encouraged by Jewish ritual killing, in conscience-tormented feeling as to Buddhist-Essene abstinence from bloodshed. People love such illusion.

In "The Works of Josephus", he is among the royalty studying with the Essenes, we find: "The Essenes (meaning

Saviors or Healers) also, as we call a sect of ours...live the same kind of life as whom the Greeks call Pythagoreans...Herod had these Essenes in such honor and thought higher of them than their mortal nature required. Now there was one of these Essenes, whose name was MANAHEM (Manaen in Aramaic meaning Gnostic knower of the Spirit of God), who had foreknowledge of future events given him by God. When Herod was a child going to school, he saluted Herod as the King of the Jews...Manahem clapped him on the back, saying, "Thou wilt be King, and wilt begin thy reign happily for God finds thee worthy of it, and remember the blows that Manahem hath given thee as being a signal of change of thy fortune...Thou wilt excel all men in happiness, obtain everlasting reputation, but wilt forget piety and righteousness and crimes will not be concealed from God, and he will punish thee for them"...Now some of the Jews thought the destruction of Herod's army came from the punishment of what he did against John called the Baptist, for Herod slew him who was a "Chrestus (Good man in Greek)...Pilate made a canal to bring water to Jerusalem, and there "was about this time, a teacher...He was the Christus (Anointed in Gk. phonetically the same as Chrestus), and when Pilate...had condemned him to the cross, those who love him did not forsake him and he appeared to them the third day...Jesus (Savior), a wise man (Gnostic) for he was a doer of wonderful works...Judas who caused the people to revolt when Cyrenius came to take an account of the estates of the Jews...The names of his sons were James and Simon, whom Alexander commanded to be crucified.....A certain magician (Magi), whose name was Theudas, who persuaded a great pact of people to take belongings and follow him to the Jordan for he told them he was a prophet and he would by his own command divide the rivers and afford easy passage over it. Fadus (procurator of Judea) did not permit it, slew many, took Theudas alive and cut off his head and carried it to Jerusalem. (When Albinus was procurator) "he assembled the Sanhedrin, and brought before them the brother of Jesus (Savior) who was called Christus (Anointed of Spirit), whose name was James, and some companions and when he had formed an accusation against James, and some companions and when he had formed an accusation against them as breakers of the Law and delivered them to be stoned...There was a man who falsely pretended, on account of the resemblances of their countenances, that he was that Alexander who was slain by Herod. He got a great deal of money,...was carried in a sedan, maintaining a royal attendance,...and received more presents in every city than ever Alexander did when he was alive. Cesar laughed at the contrivance...but put him to death." All this we quote from Josephus written 93 A.D. What caused Simon of Galilee to be crucified, in place of the Anointed Savior John (resurrected) was Josephus's testimony that he was a Zealot, and in the N.T. he used his sword to attack the soldier who came to escort Jesus away...really to royal protection. Thus the N.T. Bible states Simon of Cyrenius time or incident took the Savior's place, carrying the cross and being crucified, because in his Galilean resemblance and dialect he was identical to that of the Savior (or John). A similar earlier incident of the carrying of the head of a wonder-worker of the man on the Jordan river to Jerusalem, clearly explains how confusion in tales arose, especially encouraging Herod to enact the crucifixion and resurrection, theatrically dramatized about Alexander, in order to save John.

Also, it helped appease the rioting mobs of Jewish orthodoxy, who could only be pacified seeing bloodshed, jealous of the power of these Oriental wise men, "Prophets", Essenes, etc. The Crucifixion of Simon of Galilee fulfilled the Sacrificial "Lamb of God" tradition and prophecies, to enhance John's repeated "resurrections" prestige, and it saved the honor and sacred vow enjoined by Essenes to whom he owed all his good fortune and happiness. We have told you how Herod, Pilate, beside Josephus and Philo, contemporaries to John, from birth to Hadrian's rule (130 A.D.) all greatly honored the Gnostic Essene Savior, never revealing his whereabouts, but secretly "sub rosa" (Latin for esoterically,- "under the rose") concealing the mystery of the cross of Eastern origin. Both Herod and Pilate were reminded of their sacred Fraternal vows and made the most of the occasion to frustrate the Jewish sacerdotal opposition,-- mocking their rituals and traditions by a circus of Satire complying with the ridiculous demands,- as ever escorting John to a new territory to appear again spreading his Teachings thru-out the Near East.

Remember that Essenes means Healers or (life) Saviors, coming from the same root as "Jesus", or Savior (any one Essene), applying especially to John, as well as the Anointed of Holy Spirit title "Christ", (+) Immortal Divine Spirit. Now, reading Luke 1:78 (Rheims version), "The Orient from on High hath visited us", which for a version for Jews would be distasteful, so Matthews 1:23, he is called "Manuel" or God with us. In Samaria, John was known as the Comforter, Manaen (or Gnosis, Gnostic in Greek) with "Manaendros" (Gnostic-Man), as the Roman Church liked to pin on him, along with Simon Magus whom Rome stole their doctrines from under the title of Paul (A-Paulo, Apollo meaning "Sun" like Simon). In Antioch God with us, "Manuel", was briefly "Manaen, foster brother of Herod", in Essene form, while in Ephesius "Merinthus" (Cerinthus) writes the Revelations of Apostle John. Since the Gospel of John is only part of John's story, it could be that "+ John", Mark John or Marcion, being an Essene Bishop's son, too, like John (God-Endowed), son of bishop Zebedee's and Zacharias' son (Bestower of Apostolic Essene lineage), is the continuance of John till Hadrian's time, writing his 128 A.D. clue translation in Greek, that completes a Gnostic N.T. Gospel of St. John,- altho not personally, since Marcion differs from John in points as did Paul (Simon), altho writing under John's seal of the + (Christ).

    The Gospel warned that he who lived by the sword shall die by the sword, even John's mercy being unable to save Simon of Galilee, who was symbolically substituted for compliance with the Sacrificial Lamb myth of the deluded priests,- the founder of Gnostic Christians, Nass-Aryans or Mandaeans, Manaen being saved eternally. John, Savior Anointed in Holy Spirit "Manaen", had no fear, knowing his Immortal Karma, generated in Essene school days where he was trained along with Herod, beside the admiration Pilate had for the Essenes, made the occasion a celebration of millennial Rosicrucian mystery, now long forgotten due to man's profane mind choosing to dwell in a gory "historicity" of Crucifixion, not EXALTATION to Glory in God. As the Immortal Divine Spirit, +, unfolds, blossoming "sub rosa" in Esoteric Wisdom, we become aware only of Everlasting Life in Peace and Rejoicing of Spirit, Fearless Like Manaen, the Comforter. (The Essenes, Esoteric Rosy Cross, White Brotherhood, August Order of Living Immortals shall be traced in my coming volume of the Autobiography "MAITREYA" to the origins of the Paradisian Hyperboreans in Asia).

WHENCE:- MAITREYA, NEW AGE WORLD TEACHER, OR LOVEWISDOM AUTOBIOGRAPHY?

In the life of Gautama there came a time when sitting under a fig tree, he received True Insight, became Enlightened attaining to Sambodhi, and thus, became a Buddha. When his former followers conspired not to honor him because he violated his former first vow, giving up his ascetical practices, calling him Gautama after his family name, he replied, "Call me not after my private name for that is rude and careless in the way of addressing an Arhat. The Buddhas bring Salvation to the world and therefore they ought to be treated with respect as children treat their father." "He who looks for me, the true Tathagatha, in any material form, or sees me thru any audible sound, that man has entered an erroneous path" (Vajracchedika). "Buddhas and Bodhisattvas are not enlightened by fixed teachings, but by an intuitional process that is both spontaneous and natural" (Diamond Sutra). "Know, therefore oh Brahman, that I am the Buddha". There is no guilt in names, if one has an unknown way of Salvation, not a rehash or new arrangement, really worthy of them.

Buddha prophesied that 500 years after him another Buddha would appear. At the start of the Christian era, John the Establisher, Initiator (meaning of "Baptist" in Aramaic) founded Christianity. John's Gospel tells us, "There was a man sent from God whose name WAS John." But after John had gone to baptize or initiate disciples on the Jordan with a bathing ritual, he saw a dove rest peacefully on his head or his shoulder one day, experiencing such exaltation and illumination that he gave testimony that "I saw the Spirit coming down as a dove from heaven" that Spirit remained on him, Spiritually Anointed. Hence he gathered followers who believed he was the Anointed Savior, "Jesus Christ" in the Greek form, completely reborn as God's Spirit of Salvation. This eccentricity caused friends, relatives and followers to be concerned and thus came the rumor that John had lost his head, and disputing of former followers, who claimed he had a messiah-complex, and those who could accept that he was the prophesied Messiah. Those who knew him as born of the flesh, argued with those who believed in the Faith of the Spirit, that he was really reborn of Spirit. As the son of Zachary, the High Priest who knew Mary while she was betrothed to Joseph (as the Protevangelion confirms, altho Roman Church versions add genealogies absent in Aramaic mss.), John had the priestly authority to preach, as well as to cast out the Temple-of-Jerusalem sacrificial flesh-mongers and money-changers saying, "Make not the house of my father a house of traffic." By his own intuition, he became the Anointed Savior, beside being able to prove his Apostolic Succession by legal rights, like Sakyamuni Gautama, royal also in Buddhahood. John attributed all works to God, and his Apostles were to follow him in works and in HIS NAME. "Where two or three are gathered in my Name (Anointed Savior-Healer), there am I in midst of them."

John's Apocalypse indicates that the Spirit of the Anointed Savior shall again reincarnate 2,000 years later. On Dec. 13th 1942, Johnny Lovewisdom experienced a Spiritual Initiation, a Baptism of Heaven, receiving in him the Spirit of Avatars, Buddha and Christ, appearing to him in the clouds of Heaven gloriously, which thereupon authorized and enabled him to reveal a vast new Lovewisdom Message. He had not read any life story of Jesus, the bible, nor the life of Buddha, but henceforth he declared he was the Vehicle of the World Teacher, Buddha and Christ, confirmed by his 1945 Autobiography, altho of later curiosity he studied their lives and teachings, to be able to present the true story of his former incarnations, now perverted in myth and mockery. Intuitively he is guided so as to reveal a comprehensive New Age Encyclopedia of Vitalogical Sciences by which man would restore Paradise to earth, but also entangles the mystery of ages-old secrets as to his incarnation as to the origin of Buddhism, Christianity, and other doctrines. Other titles of this book might have been, "Hermit, Saint of the Andes and Father of the New Race and New Age", "Tibetan Yoga in the High Andes since 1942", "A Paradisian's Search for Paradise", or "MAITREYA, APOSTOLATE OF THE LIVING LOVEWISDOM STORY" which he preferred.

THE HEALING GOD SPELL OF SAINT JOHN
AND
THE APOSTOLATE OF THE LIVING LOVEWISDOM STORY
BY PATRIARCH ARCHBISHOP APOSTLE BELOVED IN CHRIST JOHNNY LOVEWISDOM

Copyright 1976 by
The Pristine Order of Paradisian Perfection
Printed and Published by
International University of the
Living Science of Man
Casilla H, Loja, Ecuador

+

+++

+

"One Jesus Christ, Indivisible
born of and in Spirit, not of
mortal flesh, crucified in all."

EPILOGUE*: THE AMAZING LOVEWISDOM REVELATION ON THE CHRISTIAN GOD-SPELL ORIGEN

"Now, there was about this time a healer, a wise man, if it be lawful to call him a man, for he was a doer of wonderful works,- a teacher of such men as receive the truth with pleasure. He drew over to him both many of the Jews and many of the Gentiles. He was anointed and when Pilate, at the suggestion of the principle men among us, had condemned him to the cross, those that loved him at first did not forsake him, for he appeared to them alive again the third day, as the divine prophets had foretold these and ten thousand other wonderful things concerning him; and the tribe of the anointed, so named from him, are not extinct at this day." From the "WORKS OF FLAVIUS JOSEPHUS", Antiquities of the Jews, Book 18, Chapter 3, Translated by William Whiston from the original in Greek, Published by S.S. Scranton Co. 1909, we have adapted our quotation as the classical bit of evidence of the historicity of Jesus Christ, other than the New Testament narratives on the legend to determine if it was

*originally an introduction, moved here due to its length and advanced topic.

entertaining fiction, or an allegorical book of philosophy such as expertly designed by Essenes, Therapeuts and Gnostics or actually a historical document. In this new work, unlike our other manuscripts, where we voice the doubt of Bible Critics as to the authenticity of this evidence in Josephus, except as an interpolation, now we shall declare a "Scriptural Holiday" by accepting the positive view, affirming that indeed this evidence actually be true, adding to a sense as to the infallible Word of All Scriptures. Does this change the evidence as to the N.T. being fiction, Allegory or History?

There is a confirmation of the above cited evidence in the same Works, Book 20 Chapter 9: "Festus was now dead, and Albinus was but upon the road; so he assembled the Sanhedrin of judges and brought before them the brother of the healer who was called anointed, whose name was James, and some others and when he had formed an accusation against them as breakers of the law, he delivered them to be stoned"... However, unlike the Whiston translation, I have used "healer" the meaning of Jesus and "anointed" as the meaning of the Greek word Christus, since, unless indicated in the text, such can be descriptive words rather than names of persons, places, etc. Christian Apologists will naturally insist they should be capitalized, but let us take the unbiast scientific viewpoint. There are even ten different Jesuses mentioned as names by Josephus, so James was the brother of whoever was called Messiah in Hebrew, or Christus in Greek or Anointed in English. Josephus finishes the paragraph saying that "King Agrippa took the high-priesthood from Ananus, and made Jesus, the son of Damneus, high priest". Then, "Jesus, son of Gamalied, became successor of Jesus, son of Damneus," and Gessius Florus became successor of Albinus! Christus or Messiah was the title of the High Priest and King, just as "Jesus" was the name of healers or saviors, coming from the verb to save just as Essene and Therapeut spoke of healers as well as the cult of Saviors among Palestinians. Josephus gives one of the most elaborate descriptions of the Essenes, beside the Jewish sects of Pharisees and Sadducees.

In his own life story Josephus states that "One whose name was Banus lived in the desert and used no other clothing than that which grew on trees and had no other food than what grew of its own accord, and bathed himself in cold water frequently both by night and by day, in order to preserve his chastity: I imitated him in those things and continued with him 3 years." He does not tell of what sect Banus was, altho he does say he did not content himself with the trials of Pharisees, Sadducees and Essenes, but took recourse to this other fourth sect. At 19, Josephus began to conduct himself according to the rules of Pharisees. At 26 he travelled to Rome with 3 priests "who supported themselves on figs and nuts, and showed piety toward God even under affliction". Then he spent many years as Governor of the Galileans and tells of encounters with Jesus, leader of a seditious tumult of mariners and poor people, setting fire to Herod's Palace and plundering the land. Also Josephus cautiously reveals a fourth sect of Jews who followed Judas a Galilean. "They have an inviolable attachment to liberty: and say God is to be their only Ruler and Lord. They also do not value dying any kind of death, nor do they heed the deaths of their relatives and friends nor can any such fear make them call any man Lord, and since this immovable resolution of theirs is well known to a great many, I shall speak no further about that matter; nor am I afraid that anything I have said of them should be disbelieved, but rather fear that what I have said is beneath the resolution they show when they undergo pain, and it was in Gessius Florus' time that the nation began to grow mad". The Jews went wild and began a revolt against the Romans. Judas' zealous sect is identified as Zealots.

Thus far, does anything told of these Galileans disagree in any way with what the N.T. Gospel of Christ teaches? Moreover, Luke 6:15, Acts 1:13, also identifies Simon as a Zealot of the Galilean's sect of what became known as Nassarenes and Christians, and Matthew 13:55 identifies Simon as the brother in this sect of James, Joseph and Judas. In Josephus' Works, Book 2 Chap. 7 of Wars of Jews, he tells of a practice of pretenders of the resurrection miracle such as a spurious one pretending to be Alexander slain by Herod, his father, and he, along with his brother Aristobulus had risen from the dead, since he greatly resembled Alexander and was instructed in his affairs, using this for the extortion of great sums of money, which greatly entertained Cesar who nevertheless put him to death. In this same book -chapter he continues telling of Simon the Essene, gifted in prophesy, just as Judas the Essene is told of elsewhere with the same gift and immediately after these individuals he tells of Judas, the Galilean of the fourth sect of Jews that started the revolt in Galilee. Josephus doesn't try to trace any of these stories but labels them by Essean, Galilean, Zealot, etc. according to opinions as to whom their acts resemble, just as today reporters label characteristic actions to certain sects.

Just as the N.T. confirms, Judas who headed the Zealots had sons or followers, James, and Simon who were crucified according to Josephus (Antiq. 20:5). This follows an explanation of the legend of "a certain Magician named Theudas persuaded a great part of the people to take their effects with them and follow him to the river Jordan, for he told them he was a prophet",- just as John the Baptist did,- and that he would by his own command divide the river and afford them easy passage over it, and many were deluded by it." Fadus stopped him, and slew many. Then he took Theudas alive, cut off his head and carried it to Jerusalem identical to what is told of John the Baptist in the N.T. Bible.

In Catholic tradition Thadeus is St. Judas, the Apostle and Brother of the Lord who wrote an Epistle of the N.T., lived as long as John the Apostle, tells of the Enoch Book of Essenes, etc. The Followers of Paul and Simon Peter quarrelled and broke up, never to meet again, so Paul's follower Luke, in Acts 5 states that Simon Peter teaches "We ought to obey God rather than men" filling Jerusalem with doctrine, beside the resurrection Savior, and then tells of Judas Theudas who resurrected or rose but they should not speak in the name of Jesus or these men. Both Judas (Theudas) and Simon (Peter) went to Mesopotamia to the Gnostic Eastern Church (Essene), after these happenings. Simon (Peter) and the Savior-Healer or Essene Christ were Crucified according to both Josephus and the N.T. Gospels, giving undeniable facts of historicity to the N.T. Bible.

When ever the historical Apostle's tales told of instances that were at all adverse, risky or condemned by the doctrines of the Roman Catholic doctrine established and first organized by St. Constantine at Nicea in 325 A.D., they were like the public opinion polls of gossip and scandal recorded by orthodox historians, as of foreigners, Gentiles, Magicians or Gnostics, Galileans, Samarians, etc. When the deeds or stories of the Apostles took on extremes but favoring the Jewish or Roman Church dogmas, they were labelled "Essene", or of a fourth sect, the "Zealots". According to Valentinus (most famous Gnostic) and Basilides, the tradition of the Apostles came with the Gnosis (Wisdom) or Holy Spirit witnessed by Theodas (according to

Valentinus, Josephus, etc.) and Matthias (according to Basilides, Acts 1 adding he was Joseph, Basabbas or Barnabas or Justus, called Judas: Acts 15) so as to round up all the authors of Palestine's tales. Naturally Thomas, author of the Gnostic Gospel of Thomas, or the "Oracles" or "Secret Sayings of Jesus", as the Twin or Spiritual Double of the Lord as Jesus' Brother Judas, Theudas, the Risen John the Baptist and Apostle combine to give mankind the First Christians of St. John in Antioch and fashioned the original New Testament God-Spell. Mysteriously, Josephus having been trained by Essene Gnostics, explains that the reason why he did not write more about the fourth sect of Judas the Galilean was because, "nor am I afraid that anything I have said of them should be disbelieved but rather fear what I have said is beneath the resolution when they undergo pain" causing Revolt to Rome, destroying Jerusalem in 70 A.D. and spreading from Galilee and Samaria to Antioch, Ephesus, Edessa, etc. this Savior's work according to Simon Peter "began from Galilee where John the Baptist preached the Gospel of Jesus of Nassareth and how he had appointed him with the Holy Spirit and with power who went about doing Good (Chrestus) and healing all that were oppressed by the devil, for God was with him" (Acts 10:38).

Now to establish our claim that Simon Magus, Magician of Samaria told of in Acts 8:9 who became a Christian and received the Apostolic power thru the laying on of hands as a follower of Phillip, and who the Roman Catholic Church accuses to be the founder of the Gnostic First Christians that turned the Eastern Church into opposition to Rome, and that these Gnostics, Magi or Magicians were precisely known also as Essenes and Therapeuts, we have the following proofs. Concerning this in Josephus' Antiquities 20:7 we read that Simon, a Jew, pretended to be a Magician (Gnostic) giving council to Drusilla to marry Felix who gave birth to Agrippa, etc. while in Book 17:13, he describes Simon the Essene interpreting a dream, (altho such sciences were of Magi and Gnostics) with stories of N.T. nature or similarity beside Archelaus divorcing his wife Mariamne also with a prophetic dream, etc. This Simon, Gnostic, Essene Magician while in Jerusalem persuaded the Jewish nation they should exclude King Agrippa from the Temple of Jews, accusing him of not living in a holy way, later described in Catholic traditions as "St. Simon of Jerusalem, a brother of our Lord". In

Catholic tradition, Simon and Judas preached in Babylonia (Mesopotamia), Judas ending in martyrdom, decapitated, identical to the head taken to Jerusalem story as told of Theudas by Josephus, beside the story of John the Baptist, while also in Catholicism it is claimed that both the remains of Simon Peter and St. Judas were taken to be placed in a crypt in St. Peter's of Rome. Likewise, Simon Peter wrote his Catholic Epistle I from the Church of the Elect in Babylon whereof he writes, altho Roman Catholic N.T. Bibles always carry a footnote, saying it is not so, rather Babylon is figurative for Rome! Encyclopedias state that St. John the Baptist's body was buried in Samaria, at the foot of Mt. Carmel, where the famous Colleges of the Carmelite Order, the Essenes and the Gnostic First Christians were founded, as well as the Samaritan Order whose God-Spell we now translate.

The foregoing description of names contemporary to Josephus and the First Century Christian Era in the N.T. Gospels, shows where the First Christians or Essene Gnostics obtained the human prototypes for their spiritualized allegories which became Christian Scriptures. As we have shown in our work "Sacred Theology of the Seven Churches of Asia" about Gnostic Christian origins of God-Spells, the First Church Fathers historically in Eastern and Western Churches both attribute that: "THOSE ANCIENT THERAPEUTS (Essenes or Gnostics) WERE CHRISTIANS AND THEIR ANCIENT WRITINGS WERE OUR GOSPELS AND EPISTLES", and Philo verifies that Therapeuts spent time in study composing and expounding these Sacred Scriptures, seeking the hidden, mystical or allegorical meaning, rather than merely adhering to historical accuracy or details in common worldly meaning. Josephus thus became the source of Jewish History that gave the original arch-types selected to illustrate symbolic, mystical or spiritual significance of the happenings in all our lives and provide means in ideals to a higher life. As the Christians preach even today, all their sins and the sins of Christian Apostles as bloody warriors, Zealots, etc. were washed away when they accept Christ nailing their sins to His cross, whose glory we sing and feast by tradition.

But some may say or ask: "But what on earth has any old Jesus myth got to do with my life after nearly two thousand years of fighting about a religion of love? Just this, that what we think about determines whether we are happy and have any ideal to live for, or whether we lose all faith in Life seeking to destroy our bodies, or become heirs to suffering thru drugs, killing, eating animals, crime, etc. The whole Roman Empire was in a Civil War started by the revolt and mystical tales of Gnostic Essenes, just as today's Governments are tumbling in corruption, with even the same scene in the Middle East. Our future happiness in what we do for a living and how we do it, is determined by better and higher ideals inspired from what kind of God-Spell, ideal or Spirit we are lead by as much as it was in John Baptist's time. Even the same sects of vegetarian controversies, how to plant or earn a living, how to eat food, treat pain, heal disease, the value of money, taxation, politics, etc. are all part of Life this moment as when Josephus admired Essenes, etc.

But what about John the Baptist? Josephus must have a lot to tell about him, having been a disciple of Banus 3 years who lived identical or perhaps was the N.T. Prototype of John the Baptist, Banus being the local term for the Bather or Baptist, like Baños is Baths in Spanish. "Now some of the Jews thought that the destruction of Herod's army came from God, and that very justly as punishment of what he did against John that was called Baptist, for Herod slew him who was a Good man and commanded the Jews to exercise virtue, both as to righteousness toward one another and piety toward God, and to come to baptism, for that the washing with water would be acceptable to him if they made use of it, not in order to the putting away of some sins, but for the purification of the body: supposing still that the soul was thoroughly purified beforehand by righteousness. Now, when many come in crowds about him, for they were greatly moved by hearing his words, Herod who feared lest the great influence John had over the people might put it into his power and inclination to raise rebellion, thought it best by putting him to death to prevent any mischief he might cause and not sparing a man who might make him repent of it when it should be too late." Antiquities 18:5.

First, this reveals why John the Baptist was the Prototype of the Savior Healer, "a wise man if it be lawful to call him a man for he was a doer of wonderful works, as a teacher of men who receive truth with pleasure...who was anointed (Christus or Messiah)...for whom Messianists or Christians are named. Take note that John is called "Chrestus" in Greek, and "Chrestos in

Latin or Good in English. Jesus defines God saying, "Why call me Good (Chrestus), One is Good (Chrestus), God." "None is Good but God." (Matt. 19, Luke 18).

In the second century, Sueton wrote about the Jewish revolt reaching Rome, caused by "impulsore Chresto (One Chrestus, like John, instigating)". Justin Martyr explained this at once, "We are Chrestians (best of men), and so it can never be just to hate what is Chrestus (Good); therefore to hate what is Chrestian is unjust." "Those that lived according to Logos were really Christians concluded the Gnostic St. Clement of Alexandria, explaining why the Word (Logos) was exemplified in Socrates, Plato, Pythagoras, etc. The Gnostic First Christians believed they were the true Messianists or Christians, which orthodox Jewish doctrine denied, except among the Essenes. Antioch thus became the Church of the Apostles that spread the God Spell (Gospel) to all other parts of the world, so that the earliest Christian Church (Marcionite) that is dated by inscription (318 A.D.) reads "The Lord and Savior (Jesus), Chrestus (Righteous)", not "Christus" or Messiah. This evidence shows that the traditional First Christians of Antioch were Gnostic Chrestians of John, the Good. The Essene Dead Sea Scrolls are shown to be dedicated to the very TEACHER OF RIGHTEOUSNESS or "Chrestus" in Greek. Even the Catholics called Judas (St. Jude), brother of our Lord or Thaddeus "the Loving" Apostle of the Lord. Simon who was a son (follower) of John Baptist (John 21) was also "son of Theodas" or Judas which Josephus tells about, identifying all the Zealots who were stopped at the Jordan River, that become Prototypes of Spiritual Rebels (that originated in John the Baptist's beheading) to Rome even. Finally, it is Judas Thomas or the Spiritual Twin, Double of the Savior that reveals the nature of the Lord, that is to say, know Christ our Healer first hand by His wounds in our flesh: "Do Penance for the Kingdom of God is at hand" being the identical words of John Baptist and Jesus. Hands and feet pierced going barefoot and weeding thistles and thorns out of Paradise, heart speared with conscience of God's Law, and head crowned with thorns of Righteousness but scorned by indignities of worldly calumny, in the wounds of Logos, Gnosis or our Inner Lord we know Him as Initiates of Christ. The Spiritual double or "Christus-Chrestus or Savior of Gnostic Chrestians in the physical body was John the Baptist, a Good man, risen as Theodus and Judas, showing the play of allegorical words of the SAME SOUND but different spelling. Thus, the Spiritual Double is purified in the Baptism of Fire in the Resurrection to the Holy Spirit, showing the Monophystic concept of Jesus Christ as Light-Fire in persons purified as John the Baptist in the physical "Temple of a Living God" or washed of sins with the Baptism of Living Water (Juicy Fruit diet) giving the Immaculate Conception without menstrual or seminal bloodshed. The Mystical allegories of the N.T. and Genesis Paradise explain today's Truth.

All the God-Spell writings of the N.T. reveal the Gnosis, which signifies Truth, Good, Love, Love or Spirit of God thru their mystical allegory spiritualizing the contemporary history of Palestine in the first and second century, along with traditional myths, just as the Gnostic Essenes had taken the gory tales of Moses, Jephtha, David, Sampson, Elijah and other war criminals who slaughtered thousands, beside the bloody sacrifices of innocent harmless sheep, doves and other animals on Jewish alters in Temple worship, denying their value before God, participating only in unbloody offerings to God and mystically interpreting sacrifice as the overcoming of our animal natures and sin. The Spirit of Jesus (Saviors) is Indivisible, One in all who live in Him.

People who read the N.T. Bible taken outside of the Jewish history of old Palestine in the first century are generally shocked at the cruelty and the mockery of the crucifixion story. If they would insert the story of the N.T. Jesus Christ in with the rest of all the gory tale, where crucifixions and the setting up of all kinds of ignoble traitors (some of whose names were also Jesus) and making mockery of Jewish tradition about the Anointed Priest-Kings in a recurrent sadist circus, who would want to be part of any Anointed-King Son of David the champion of War Criminals and assassins? With all the fraud Josephus tells of miracle-pretenders of his day, one would easily suspicion such claims for a man of virtue and holiness. People are finally beginning to question the integrity of Kings who claim God is on the side of Killers and criminals who attack peaceful people in aggressive wars. Only if we understand the Crucifixion story as a mystical initiation in allegorical symbolism is its true worth discovered. The vicarious atonement of animals never saved man from his sins, and much less the killing of any human scapegoat sacrificed, as Christians now claim. People should read Josephus and see for themselves.

Luckily, I was not overwhelmed by Jesus' crucifixion, when I first read the N.T. Bible in 1944. However I was mystically awakened, with tears running down my cheeks as I read about John the Baptist who lived so close to my ideals at that time as a hermit, and yet was beheaded for the Truth he preached, just as in my work "Lessons from the Life of Love-Wisdom" or my 1945 Autobiography I described my former reincarnations, including living before as John the Baptist. Thus, I have realized my Spiritual Return, or Resurrection of John, as the Eternal Apostle Beloved in Christ. My early background with a conscience against bloodshed and killing, in my first journal at Lake Quilotoa Sept. 13, 1946, I began preaching, "For nearly 2,000 years the world has lived in the Passion of Jesus, martyrs, crusades, stigmas and all the bloody manifestation: He said he brought the sword and not peace. It was a necessary Purification. Instead of the horrible passion scenes, I bring mankind the Message and Gospel of the Eternal Youth Life, a Profound Peace to abide in a Divine Race..." Pain only punishes personal errors in ignorance, ignoring Truth, till the Spirit is purified to Godhood. As the Gospels label them, the Virgin Birth, the Living God-Spell and the Resurrection are all Spiritual Initiations, but the Crucifixion was intended to awaken in mankind an abhorrence to war crimes and the Slaughterhouse Temples the Jews had made their religion. Surely, I felt that a Just God of Love would not punish a true Healer-Savior without any blemish in sin. So like other Gnostic-Chrestians, even while training as a Catholic Carmelite, I believed and taught that somehow Jesus escaped suffering, or just as he had created food out of thin air to feed 5,000, the Crucifixion was all a hypnotic delusion of no physical substance, leaving no remains in his tomb, and that the Christ was a Spiritual Double that could pass thru locked doors. He was the Light, Life and Love of God. The Gospels (Matt. 27:32, Mark 15:21, Luke 23:26) say Simon of Cyrene took the cross and was crucified, which is a key to the whole allegory, since Simon was the son of Judas, Theudas, or the founder of Zealot revolutionaries, as Josephus told it historically when Cyrenius took over Syria-Palestine, giving the Simon of Cyrenius era label in the N.T. allegory. Pilate had it in his power to rescue a sinless God-man but the bloodshed of warriors never escapes punishment, no matter how righteous man claims any cause. The mystical Body and Blood of Christ is Indivisible, all-One.

As Philo of Alexandria and Josephus both have explained, The Essenes, etc. originated in Central Asia, while the historic introduction of Buddhist Yogis, or Gymnosophist missionaries into Syria-Palestine and Egypt, teaching non-violence and vegetarianism beside reincarnation and deeper Spiritual doctrines of Gnostics, all came with Alexander's kingdom extending to India, and the resulting exchange of Culture favoring the Pythagorean philosophy. Philo identifies the Therapeut Essenes as Wisdom-Lovers or Philo-Sophers, those who Love Wisdom, as the true Healing God-Spell and Living Lovewisdom shall reveal more on now. The key to Christ's Kingdom is that the Savior, Jesus, is Indivisible, as flesh is.

Simon Magus of Samaria to whom the Roman Church attributes their cause for weakness and lack of faith in other Christians to originally, they hold to be a First Gnostic Christian who was a follower of John the Baptist, and mystically is identical to Simon Peter and Simon, the Brother of the Lord, is identical to Simon of Gitta. This curious evidence, revealing more of the Hindu Bible, the Bhagavad Gita, and the origins of Mahayana Buddhist Yoga of High Tibet and the Himalayas in contribution to their Scriptures dated as recorded in the first Christian Century, as well as Kristna becoming the Kristus whose Jnana or Wisdom Yoga becomes the Gnosis of mystical "Oracles" or Sayings of the Savior (Jesus), but with Syria-Palestine historical names taken as symbols in meaning. So the Palestine battlefields become the Dharma Kcheta or Kurukchetra of the senses, as symbolized in the Gita. Simon is the cornerstone upon which the Church or Ecclesia is Founded, for which reason Rome and the Popes have valued traditions of Apostolic Faith. Beside conceding to name him as the Great, Simon Magus, he is the "doer of wonderful works" or Jesus-Healer that Historian Josephus tells about, which Acts 8:10 says "to whom they all gave ear" in Samaria the Essene-Carmelite-Gnostic Center teaching the Living Water (John 4:10) doctrine of John Baptist Christians. Now the "Metaphysical Bible Dictionary" of Unity School founded by the great vegetarian leader, Charles Fillmore explains that "Simon means one who listens and obeys". Peter is the word meaning rock or stone, or the kind of firm Faith one must build one's Ecclesia (assembly) of ideals upon. On this Faith Christ built his Ecclesia and power of is-ness Thou art Christ, or the "I AM" Consciousness gives control of the Heavens or the "Keys to the Kingdom of the Heavens" (Matt. 16:19). "I and the Father are One...Ye are Gods...God's Kingdom of Heaven is within". But Jesus said we must never reveal or tell anyone who He really was, the Judas of Galilee of Josephus history and Simon Zealot, his Crucified Brother. (Matt. 16:20, Acts 5:40). However, this Church Cornerstone or Petros can fall into error and become a scandal and stumbling stone, so "get thee behind me Satan", He tells Simon (Matt. 16:23, 21:42). That is because Steadfastness of Faith (Petros) is only developed thru Love (John Apostle Beloved in Christ) as Simon is the son of John Baptist (see John 21:15-23) so that John shall remain till Christ has come. This Resurrected John of the Heavenly Ecclesia, under his seal, embrace or laying of hands in Patriarch Archbishop Lovewisdom has united the Western Catholic and Eastern Gnostic Orthodox Faiths, including all Christians, as well as the Spiritual Head Lama (Tashi) and all the Sects of Buddhism and Hindu Yoga, as well as Sufi, Taoist, and all others as explained since 1945, - see "A Cosmic Universal Conception of the Holy Life". Even the Popes of Rome by claiming infallibility in 1870 have erred giving the Apostolic Catholic Succession to the Old Holy Catholic Church, just as the immature boy placed in the Dalai Lama office before legal status of Lamas, returned the Head of the Heavenly Hierarchy to its origin in the Tashi Lama, which was secretly transferred to the Andes and in Righteousness vested with the Father of the New Race and New Age of Paradisians (Homo Paradisicus). Henceforth, with God's Grace Waves THE PRISTINE ORDER OF PARADISIAN PERFECTION shall guide the earth and mankind and save all Life from complete chaos or destruction, altho there is much more pruning and purification necessary. Often it will seem contradictory or lost in confusion, when we have affirmed Truth in Roman Catholic, Buddhist or any other of dozens of doctrines at our disposal, but mystically in our Telepathic Gnosis in Holy Spirit and Truth Love-Wisdom shall be found in the Heart and Mind of all who seek. Simon listens and obeys for firm Faith thru John Be-Love...d.

Religion has the same meaning as Yoke or Yoga, since thru it we Re-League with God for Re-Legion, which requires Integrated Knowledge or Wisdom in God, the Integrity of Gnosis. The Integrated God Spell, or Cosmic Consciousness, gives Logos or His Word which is discovered in the Canonical Bible combined with the Gnostic Bible of Essenes, etc. beside an insight into the Bibles of Buddhists, Yogis, etc. Seeing that only 3 times has the Bible ever mentioned the word "Christian", at first being usually in contempt for this Messianist sect, altho they were often named to be Nass-Aryans, or Nass-Arius (Arius is a Gnostic who held that only after the Baptism of John did Jesus become a Christ, as now said of Christians). Nassarene is used often by its Apostles or Gnostics. In fact numerous writers have shown that Nassaret did not exist at the time of the first century N.T., which instead was really a synonym for Galilee where the Jesus legends are centered. All this relates to the term "Nass" which means Serpent, first told of in Eden as to who tempted Eve to eat of the forbidden fruit which brought sexual passion to mankind. Thus, the First Chrestian sect to deal with the Kundalini Serpent Force of the Essene tradition was called Nass-Essenes or Nassenes, in which the Paradise-Regained or Heaven-Realm of Consciousness is restored turning the Jordan and the 4 Streams of Eden (Sight, Hearing, Smell, Taste) back to their Source. Thus, true Christians were anointed with the "Ineffable Chrism" poured out by this Serpentine Horn of Plenty (Cornucopia) by Sublimating the Sexual Powers giving rise to Spiritual Rebirth and Enlightenment or the Gnosis. Ophite, Nass-Aryan or Nass-Essene sects of Gnostic Christians with Yoga (Arya-India) doctrines had Scriptures which say Jesus turned the waters of the Jordan to flow back to its Source (Snow on Mt. of Transfiguration, Hermon, Zion, as well as Golgotha or skull place in the body). Each region of Jordan, Jesus of the God-Spell told in the N.T. Bible is the region of miraculous powers therein described, just as Yogis in India reverse the flow of the Ganges back to the Himalayan Heights of snow-white God-Consciousness. Like Christus and Chrestus of the same sound but with multiple meanings, the Gnostic Greek term, in Aramaic dialects was related to Nass-Teaching even tracing origins to Sethians below Eden snows on Mt. Hermon (as told of in the Book of Adam and Eve, preaching a strict fruit diet). "Be ye wise as Serpents, and harmless as doves" and lifting up the Serpent in the Wilderness like Moses (Jn. 3:14) is a strictly Nass Aryan doctrine of the Buddhist Yogis.

Hate kills and destroys, giving wars. Love heals, builds and gives Peace to all. The Healers of nations shall love even the sick minds bent on war, who became sick by generations of prejudice, jealousy and hate preached even today in the name of Religions of Love. Those who preach fear of things anti-Christ, anti-Semetic, anti-Aryan, anti-Russian, anti-American, or even anti-Anti are still preaching hate, illusion, fear which can only be healed by Love-actions. The Essenes were admired because even tho they hated wrong actions in slaughterhouse cults and wars, they took the symbolic allegorical meaning of Scriptures in names or terms, that were assembled into legends to teach virtue, love or truth.

If one has always regarded Jesus as a flesh and bones person, and not the Highest Light, Love and Life of a mystical body or Ecclesia known thru the Holy Spirit, it will be hard to realize the Gnostic Logos can manifest in all times, anywhere and in anyone really seeking Him. Yet, thus he travelled with those First Christians of John, who did not just get ceremonial washing in the Jordan, consoling their spirits, but instead were fired by the Light of the World he gave out in his Life sustained by wild carob (locust-beans) and honey, enough to follow him in the Holy Spirit. These followers spread miracles of healing thru-out Palestine and the world in the Anointed Savior's Name thru Love. His Name is Good, Chrestus, or John (Loving-Grace), which saves (Jesus) and thus becomes Christus (Messiah) which is Immanuel (within you). In summary we have shown how N.T. Names were historic names, but cleansed from warrior and sinner personality working their freedom out by Love of both Jewish and Roman oppressors, just as today we must face and realize in our modern world.

"Catholic bishops and teachers know not how better to stem this flood of Gnostic Scriptures and their influence among the faithful, than by boldly adopting the most popular narratives from the heretical books, and after carefully eliminating the poison of false doctrines, replacing them in this purified form in the hands of the public," writes one of the most authoritive orthodox writers, Lipsius, explaining how even the accepted N.T. Bible came into being. If one will note, nobody can for sure say who the authors that wrote each of the Gospels and Epistles were, these names being added or assigned to each book only by tradition, as the Confraternity Catholic Bible now admits rightly, nor could they have put their own names to them, because such writings were by law forbidden in their time under death penalty.

Kreyenbuhl's exhaustive study, claims an immediate origin for the FOURTH GOSPEL, which is the most Spiritual one of all, as none other than the Gnostic Menandros, a native of Samaria and the earliest active teacher in Antioch who was the teacher of Basilides, and who Justin claimed to be famous because of his numerous following. Also known as Meandros, it leads his teaching to be considered the origin of Mandeans, or Gnostic Magi of Samaria, later surviving as Manicheans, vegetarians who refused even milk and eggs with Buddhist tendencies awaiting Maitreya the Buddha. He claimed the Savior was Logos and that man might so perfect himself that he becomes a conscious worker of Logos, all those who did so became Christs and such were Saviors just as he had achieved Saviorhood. Realizing a certain state of interior purification or inner enlightenment, is to "rise from the dead" and therefore "never grow old" and become Immortal possessing an unbroken consciousness of the Higher Spiritual Self. Peculiar as First Gnostic Christians of John, Meandros was possibly the Teacher of Simon the Great Wonder Worker, and another Gnostic, Dositheus, who both were followers of John the Baptist, allied to the Essenes, likewise in claiming to be incarnations of the Great Power. They set up the system of Aeons (Avatars, Buddhas, Saviors) of Gnostic doctrines, the Heavenly Man with 7 and 12 planets, etc. or Powers around the Central Sun, the meaning of the word Simon. Later we shall quote Gnostic writings on the Gnosis of Simon (sun, male, great power and Fire) dwelling in man as Logos, or the temple of the Holy Spirit, in their romance with Helen (moon, female, Sophia, Maria, etc.) generating or building the symbolic Tree-Man, that bears golden juicy fruit like tiny spherical suns for communion in Living Water bearing Fire in Cosmic Consciousness divinizing man. Unfortunately very little was allowed to survive from these great men who gave our N.T. Holy Bible, because the Catholic Church Fathers were most concerned in weeding out their heresies, filling their biographical data on Gnostic First Christians with details correcting supposedly their errors and condemning exaggerated falsehoods, for the "fathering" of a truly "inspired Word of God", feeling thus they could return their Scriptures to public circulation, while denying they were really the true authors, so as to give credit to historic Zealots contemporary to the allegorical "Jesus Christ".

Not only could Men-andros, Meandros, etc. (changing from Samarian, Syriac to Greek eventually) have been the founder of Mandeans (Manda means Gnosis), as well as Mani who is said to have given the First Christian doctrine to Manicheans, but later he lived at Ephesus as Merinthus, otherwise called Cerinthus by Irenaeus. Altho Irenaeus sought to hide the true author by stating, "John wrote his Gospel to confute the doctrines of Cerinthus", this denial shows who the real author among the doctrinal "heretics" to Rome's Church was. In fact, Irenaeus is the first person to name authors to the four gospels, which like four winds and seasons blow immortality into man, developing Rome's law or canon on authorized Scriptures and assigning allegorical evangelists as the true authors. Irenaeus thus worked John's Gospel over, stealing what he did write, and claiming contrary to popular knowledge and evidence from Cerinthus what the Roman Church censored "heretical". Likewise, well known was the fact that, as Gnostics had proven, that Cerinthus was the author of the Apocalypsis or Revelations of John, so as to be omitted from canon often, but containing Cerinthus' own denial of any association with Nicolaitans (who ate animal flesh and fornicated yet claiming they were Gnostic-Christians, Apoc. 2:15), beside characterizing the power-mad Roman Church as the Harlot of Babylon due to the flesh-eating doctrines of Paul, Luke and misleading Peter even, against the pure Essene principle of John and other Gnostic Chestians, condemning claims by Irenaeus. This Gnostic Essene controversy with Roman Heretics broke the Christian Church in halves, the original Eastern and legalized Western bodies.

Altho the First Epistle of John could well be of Gnostic inspiration, the second and third Epistles even the Church Historian Eusebius doubted, as their content reveal, claiming the teacher of Polycarp who assumed the title of the Presbyter John to be their author. Irenaeus uses his "Life of Polycarp" to dramatize his dirty tales against Gnostic First Christians of the East, such as when Presbyter John had once entered a bath in Ephesus, seeing Cerinthus already in the bath, he was supposed to have said, "Let us leave at once lest the roof fall asunder, now that Cerinthus, the enemy of truth is in this bath!" Also, Polycarp is accused of the tale that when Marcion "chief of heretics" had approached him asking, "Do you happen to know me", Polycarp being told by companions, had replied "I know, I know, you are the son of Satan!" Likewise, the overwhelming popularity of Valentinus, another Gnostic and Gospel writer, all frustrated Roman rulership, so small wonder that Rome took to force to become the Capital of Christiandom, and the center of hundreds of spicy traditions invented against Gnostic First Christians, Zealots and Jealous rulers of all.

Finally, last in this same Johannine problem (involving enough data for a book) is the Evangelist, Mark John, author of the SECOND GOSPEL of the N.T. who was Marcion (Marc-Ion, Mark John) the Gnostic Bishop of Pontus. His disciples were rigid ascetics, abstaining from marriage, all flesh foods and wine, but otherwise ardent defenders of the original tradition of Simon Peter's Gnostic Gospel on which Paul preached at Pontus, that Christ is meaningless in the flesh and known wholly by his Spiritual nature as Paul had experienced. Thus, Marcion's large following among First Christians held that Christ, or the Jewish Messiah in traditional Jewish mockery of the sadist story of Golgotha or Calvary was the lie, and as we mentioned the earliest dated Chrestian Church of the Marcion following at Antioch. Marcion even sorted out in parallel columns what could be accepted and what was to be condemned in the Old Testament, as to what was of Good (Chrestos), just and holy God, and what must be rejected about the Mean, Jealous and Vengeful Jehova of Slaughterhouse-Temple Jews. The Aramaic Gospel of Paul used at Pontus was evidently that of Simon Peter, still in existence teaching that the resurrected Jesus extended from earth to sky, etc. which Marcion translated into Greek, and thus he had to explain to Tertulian, being of Paul, Simon Peter, etc. he could not put his name to it, altho Tertulian taunted him for showing that he wrote it beside saying he pirated some of its passages from Luke (appearing after his mss.), since the facts presented came from Paul and Simon Peter. However, in the end, he joined the Gnostic Essene Christians, whom the Roman Church forced into exile into Babylon (supporting the interpolations of Paul and Luke defending meat-eating, marriage, etc.), against Early Church vegetarianism, as Peter's Epistles and Acts of the N.T. state. Altho Marcion converted more followers to Christianity thru-out the Graeco-Roman "world" than Roman Catholicism of his time, after the first Ecumenic Councils his vegetarian, frugal spiritually oriented bishops were gradually replaced with the power-mad meat-eating church dictatorship followers of Rome.

Similar to these unscrupulous piratings to obtain the official canonical New Testament from Gnostic Essene Christians, was the case of MATTHEW'S GOSPEL written by Basilides. This

Gnostic Christian Philosopher of Alexandria, held that he was Gaucia's disciple who was an interpreter of Simon Peter of whom Matthias received the teachings in secret after the Resurrection as the Sayings or Oracle of the Lord Jesus Christ underlying all the Synoptic Gospels. Not only was Basilides the first and most learned Old Testament and Christian Exegete (exegist), but like St. Clement of Alexandria and Origen he taught reincarnation and the Law of Karma, and thus established the Gospel's allegorical interpretation that Jesus never deserved or was actually crucified on the cross but was substituted for by Simon of Cyrene. (Just as Josephus recorded that Simon, son of Juda of Galilee in Cyrenius era, as Luke 2:2 affirms also, was the Zealot actually crucified, and thus is the celebrated warrior whom Christianity now honors as suffering for all of the world's sin, once and for all!) Beside this unwavering Faith in Virtue, and logic that Sinless Godhood in our Lord, he also imposed a 5 year's silence on his disciples, held marriage was natural and not Church property, revealed the mysteries of the Ogdoad or Uncreated Father of Gnosis who Jesus received in Baptism, taught deep Mahayana Buddhist doctrines of Naught or Void as the origin of all, all of which included and continued in the above mentioned traditions of Mandeans or Gnostic Church of John.

In turn for LUKE'S GOSPEL of the N.T., much has been borrowed from Peter's Gospel beside others and especially the Protevangelion of James the First Christian Bishop of Jerusalem, ignoring or allegorically interpreting the part which states the father of Mary's child was Zacharias, who knew her as an undefiled virgen in the Temple, and immediately she heard the Holy Spirit tell her she would conceive and bring forth a child, which her cousin Elizabeth consented to take care of as her own Lord, since she was barren, and thus gave the Gnostic allegory of the mystical Virgin Birth which Jew's held illegitimate otherwise. John the Baptist was the name of the carnal vehicle that became the son of Zacharias and the barren Elizabeth, while for the N.T. Gospel in the Savior or "Jesus" meaning, he was a child by the Gnosis or Holy Ghost of Mary betrothed to Joseph, appearing to John while baptizing in the Jordan, and became the Christ or mystical body of the Church Faith after the Resurrection. Making the Gnostic Scriptures illegal under penalty of death, so there was no legal way to claim them, while the writers had championed one another combining the historical legends and tallest tales evading physical realities of life so as to enthrone an Infallible Mystic Spirit in the Christ that no other Pagan doctrine could imitate, eventually gave Rome the choice and most attractive consensus of public approval in the canonical Scriptures. Rather than avoid the Nicolaites tradition, or the "Gospel of Judas" (of Zealots, Cainites, etc.) who pretended meat eating, unlimited procreation, etc. were not evils Essenes had objected to, the Roman Church realized the profit such weaknesses in men could be exploited for very early introducing Sacraments remedying such evils from birth to death. Laboring with this condition of events already in the first 80 years of the second century A.D, Valentinus was known to compose one of the Gospels seeking outwardly to be the most "Catholic" of contemporaries, this could be no other than that of Luke. Like the Church later, he invented the position condemning the two natures of Christ (Virgin Born flesh and Spirit) and holding the concept that Christ worked out his own Divinity as to being One in all his nature. Valentinus named Theodas or Judas or St. Jude (of Josephus and Roman Church) the traditional Apostle of Mesopotamia and Africa, as to who secretly taught him the Gnosis after the Resurrection which no one could comprehend which he gave out in his Luke Gospel. He always remained outwardly a loyal Catholic all his life, and claiming Jesus ate so little and digested all so as to have no waste thru his power of continence, showing ideals he lived by, this doctrine may have inspired Early Desert Fathers of the Church as well as becoming the prototype of the Race of the "Elect" of the Heavenly Church which standards for canonized Saints were established by. In fact, to this day, St. Valentine's Day is the most celebrated by the public from Early Church fact altho now the Roman Church denies Valentinus, the Greatest of Gnostic First Christians had anything to do with its doctrine. This mystic's doctrines that was later found to have been the author of the Sophia Mythus, geometrized Ogdoad and Pythagorean and Platonic systems of syzygy concepts of Pleroma and aeonology, quietly he was excommunicated even with his place in Heaven.

Thus, the doctrines of Pagans, Jews, Greeks, Buddhist Yogis and Magi were all assimilated to give the most super-natural, miraculous and Incredible-but-True doctrines for the Mystical Body of Christ or Church. At the Council of Nicea, 325 A.D. this

Creed became law and held that "The Holy Catholic and Apostolic Church anathemizes those who say there was a time when the Son of God was not...or is created, changeable or alterable." We cannot deny such standards of Godhood when understood were high, but they also were perverted in every way to persecute competitive teachers, and yet in their own fold upholding the purloined Gnostic Christian theology without their discipline in their clergy. In all, the Essenes had woven together in the allegorical N.T. Gospels dozens of gory narratives, too awful to tell the true nature of. In one of these told by Josephus, just before the final destruction of the Temple in Jerusalem, Mary of Bethsub or Bethany beyond the Jordan, who in intolerable famine where people had begun to eat leather, etc. in her passion roasted her own child rather than let it become only a slave to Romans if it lived, eating half and hiding the other half, and when the seditious smelled her food, she gave them the remaining portion saying: "This is my own be-gotten son: Take eat this food of my body as I have eaten of it: Do you pretend to be more tender than woman, more compassionate than a mother,"- which surprisingly fits into the teaching of the Holy Eucharist where Christ offers his body flesh and blood for communicants to partake in, which no one would want to take in a full literal sense. Gnostic Essene allegories reveal it really means that the Savior will never return till in the Rule of Good (Chrestus) God's Kingdom as in Paradise we partake only of the Living Water fresh in Juicy Fruits as the purifying baptismal water exclusively and perpetually as the banquet of the Lord. Using the obvious Truth of such Gnostic First Chrestian doctrines, but practicing the promotion of alcoholic drink and pasty bread rationed to hungry slaves to quell constant upheaval provoked by hate, fear, anger and jealousy the Holy Roman Church-Empire prospered till Science gods busted out so as to leave the world spiritually lost, but ready for the new Lovewisdom Message.

    In his Preface of the 1937 original version of THE ESSENE GOSPEL OF JOHN Prof. Edmond Bordeaux Szekely stated he published only a fragment, about an eighth of the complete gospel which exists in Aramaic in the Library of the Vatican and in Ancient Slav in the Royal Library of Hapsburg". He followed that with a promise, "An edition containing the complete text with all the necessary references and explanatory notes is at present in preparation." Nearly 40 long years have sped by, and yet he was unable to trace or translate the Complete Gospel, now brushing it aside with the frank opinion of Aldous Huxley that his Book II of the Essene Gospel was only suited as "a cure for insomnia", - since when one tries to read it he falls asleep! His first edition was excellent, presenting the most obvious and avoiding frailties of the Full Gospel.

God's will had it another way: We made our first attempt to visit Prof. Szekely the year after his publication came out, but he was reported to have left his Lake Elsinore, California residence I later lived at also, while a few years later at the Temple of Meta Aum (L. Quilotoa) I translated his 1942 Edition on brown paper into Spanish, having now spent over a generation of Life molded in this ideal of higher Gnostic Chrestian Interpretation of the Healer (as Jesus means) of Mankind, enabling the Parallel Life Story of Spiritual Initiations which will be revealed with a Complete "HEALING GOD-SPELL OF JOHN". The new title translation may surprise some, but may I add in our natural frankness that in Aramaic there are no capitals or small letter distinctions, and names, unless otherwise indicated, may be translated as words. "Jesus" means Healer, including Savior of Nations, but there is no indication in such terms whether they are of spiritual or physical nature. Healers are Therapeuts or Essenes (Iessaei), while their God-Spell is thus Healing or Saving lives. God Spelle we use because the Anglo-Saxon root "God Spelle" means just that, and not "Good News" etc. as Bible-Christians often preach. "Spelle" (Chamber's Eng. Dict.) means "any form of words supposed to possess magical power; to be cast into a spelle is to be in a trance", so actually it indicates the God-Entrancement Initiation. John is a name of men but otherwise means God's Grace, God-Given or God-Endowed manifesting Love.

Most of my readers read my works because my health and natural life teaching combines with it a spiritual interpretation or deeper meaning, nor does it seek to save the sensuous physical body, or merely preach soul-saving. Many rebel, if not detest mixing health and spiritual subjects, either unable to tolerate or accept the physical or mystical natural to balanced minds, but we are not concerned with special phobias on either side. We love all and teach all, so both the Healing God-Spell and Living Lovewisdom story will contain both interpretations. The actual

Healing God Spell of John is one of the oldest and most modernly complete Natural Healing textbooks, so with our introduction to the Gnostic Chrestian origins of the New Testament Scriptures, we have synthesized Hermetical, Magi, Sufi, Buddhist-Yoga, Essene-Therapeutic teachings in a Cosmic Vision (or given time) a Compendium for a University doctorate education. Prof. Szekely described it partially in his Comotherapy.

In "First Principles", Herbert Spencer claimed to give the general discovery of the Theory of Evolution years before Darwin, which contains the interesting remarks about primitive assumption or claims of monarchs, rulers and religious leaders and authorities for which they were worshipped as Gods of Celestial Origin, or having divine rights, powers and authority, which has ironically become the position that Science assumes and claims on human life on this planet today. Science is the King, the God, explaining all and doing all without question almost. Kings reduced all men to slaves like beasts, but now Science classifies man with chattering monkeys or baboons and assumes the moronic belief that Creation came together without any need of an intelligent Divine Author because of the Universal Law of Chaos simply with a Big Bang beyond statistical chance. Neither as a Scientist nor as Spiritual Leader, have I assumed mystical knowledge for lack of Scriptural study or Divine Grace and authority for powers of their qualification. Nor have I assumed any kind of superiority in psychological balance by ignoring the damaging evidence or proof as to whether I am, or not, just a religious fanatic raving about my experience or insight, since I am very capable of labeling the phobias, manias or complexes of typical psychoanalytical or psychiatric minds.

My life in Ecuador has made three of my homesites world famous locations, contrary to wanting to be bothered by tourists. In this work I hope to show evidence or give the necessary source where one may witness for themselves facts about what I claim or assume such as: (1) Rather than out of chance, personal endeavor or assuming titles, out of God's Grace I have been endowed with renown world-wide in 1942 as the FATHER OF THE NEW RACE, Age and Order of Paradisians, followed by world-wide publicity reaching 100 million as a Hermit SAINT OF THE ANDES in 1949, beside World Spiritual Leadership in combined direction of Eastern and Western Christianity as well as Buddhist Yogic doctrines for my Mission of guiding mankind and this earth out of chaos and death throes that now threaten us, and all this a GENERATION before all of the would-be messiahs, seers, etc. marketing their wares today. Actually I will produce evidence that thru Telepathic Grace Waves of Love emanations as often claimed for Mahatmas and other Heads of a Heavenly Hierarchy or Great White Brotherhood that I initiated in operation a generation ago, today's young people have physically changed and are being modeled in religious trends and emotional rebellion to past standards of what was believed cultured civilization. My books as they are distributed more widely will continue the establishment of this New Race, New Age, New Order of Paradisians and Paradise on earth.

(2) In world-wide acceptance in Scientific Research my studies have led science to two more most famous discoveries in America, making the last two locations I lived at in Ecuador world famous. At Otavalo, living with Indians of a most ancient advanced origin, my home was a short distance from the excavation site of the oldest fossil remains of man in America, confirmed internationally by my vegetarian friend, Dr. David Davies, leading London University medical text writer on anthropology, degenerative diseases, etc., later followed by his confirmation of facts I first brought out about numerous centenarians at Vilcabamba which early in the 1960's, I began promoting as the "Sacred Valley of Longevity". These findings were confirmed in turn by Dr. Alex. Leaf head of Harvard University Medical School, who had graduated and taught at the Univ. of Wash. at Seattle, after I rejected my parents support of a medical career to teach the world vegetarianism, only to end up at Vilcabamba, which in National Geographic magazine etc. Dr. Leaf compared with Caucasus and Hunza as areas of the highest longevity average on earth,- 1973. My appearance on Television thru-out the U.S., Germany, England, Spain, Brazil, etc. concluded a Generation of world-wide publicity about my 1940 "SEARCH FOR PARADISE."

Finally, the Ecuadorian Government incorporated the "Pristine Order of Paradisian Perfection" in 1975, approving our use of our natural Vitalogical Sciences for the healing of physical and mental ailments, and other teachings. Our Order of Paradisian pioneers wishes you "Happy God Entrancement and Health".

INDEX

A-Braham (Braham) 153, 158
Abel 45
Abscesses 70, 72
Acts of Apostles 33
Affirmations 45
Age, Spiritual New 3, 147
Agape 40
Aggressiveness 94
Alexandrian Library 1
Allegories 9, 11, 31, 54, 56, 176
Adam 21, 92
Air (Angel) 36, 110, 124
(food) 124
Alkahest 114
Alcohol 34, 40, 100, 102, 103
Altar 118
Amenorrhea 29, 93
Angels of Heaven 110, 111
Angel of Pain 19
Anointed One 12, 14, 15
Anointing balsam 116
Anointed Apostles 104
Angel of Hunger 120
Animals (clean) 98
Apollos (A-Paulo) 30
Apostles 104, 131
Apostolic Creed 85
Apostolic Succession 31, 167
Appetite 126
Archives (Living) 133
Arteries 127
Atonement (vicarious) 176
Attitude of Gratitude 121, 123
Augustine 161
Autobiographic
Compendium 158
Avocado 128, 148
Avatar 149
Ballast 102
Banana 128
Banus, Banim Fw., 158, 169
(*) Fw. FOREWORD abbreviated
above, or before page 1

Bardesanes 82, 161
Baptism 37, 39, 40
Baptist (Initiator) 14
Basilides 33, 161
Baur 30
Beasts 98
Bethany Fw.,* 155
Beelzebub 19
Beloved (David) 90, 153
Biology 74
Blessings 20, 68
Blavatsky 149
Blood 20, 53, 159
Black Magicians 71, 72, 105
Bliss 62
Boils 20
Bones 17 (brittle) 127
Book of Life 63
Bonner (Joseph) 90, 151, 156
Brain 70, 74
Brahmachayra 158, 161
Braham 28, 153
Brothers 45
Bread (food) 40, 111, 112, 113
Book of Dead 7, 97
Brotherhood,
Great White Fw., 5, 52, 96
Buddha 51, 91, 126, 158
Buddhahood 156, 159
Buddhist-Yogis 108, 156, 158
Business, exploiting
disease as 76
Cain 95
Camels Fw., 91, 109
Carob Fw., 110
Carmel 28
Cells 67, 69, 70, 71, 72, 74
Catholic bishops 181
Clement of Alexandria 175
Clay jars, mss. in 1
Chewing of food 116

Character in food 125, 126
Ch'An 142
Chenrezi Lind 147, 149, 150
Chinning on bar 125
Chakras 56
Christna, Kristna Fw., 160, 178
Chrestians 175, 177
Christian, 3 times in N.T. 180
Christ potential 2
Christ - see cross
Clabber 95
Cleanser of cells 127
Church of Rome 14, 74, 87, 108
Compassion 133
Complete version 2
Commandments of Nature 22
Cooking Fw., 106
Continence 34, 39, 56
Corpulent body 124
Covering of food 116
Cornerstone 159, 178
Council of Nicea 85, 158
Cradle of New Race 179
Co-worker of God 64
Creator 23
Creed, Apostolic (600 AD) 85
Commandments of God 92, 98
Crime 19, 132
Criminal physicians 77
Criminals 93, 125
Crucifixion 24, 25, 158
Cry in Wilderness 152
Cross 158, 159, 160
Cycles 3, 99, 102
Daniel 104
Death process 142
Dead Sea Scrolls 175
Death 109
Dead Bread 111, 115
Dead food 109
Defence cells 70

Dear 150
Degeneration 75
Didache 39, 123
Dharma Kaya 54
Disease as business 76
Diseases 20, 75
Digestion 115, 123
Digestive tract 117
Discipline 142, 143
Diatessaron 161
Dried fruits, veg., 111
Dollinger 97
Drugs 69-73, 101, 131
Drug mongers 71
Earth (Angel) 64
Earthy Mother 16
Eating to live 122, 126
Eating in excess 121, 126
Excess Weight 102, 124
Eating wrong 129
Ecuador 88
Eden 92
Edessa 159, 161
Egyptian Mysteries 7, 161
Egypt 111
Elemental Spirits 124
Elimination 37, 42, 56
Elephants 109
Elias (Elijah) 14, 27, 156
Enemas 38, 55
Enzymes 111
Emotions 120, 125
EPILOGUE 168
Escape seeking 131
Essenes 97, 157, 158, 178
Essene Gospel of John 87, 77
Evangelio de Salud
de San Juan 4, 147
Eyes 42, 43
Eunuchs 39, 158
Eucharist 40, 187

Exalt (means crucify) 24, 159
Evils of world 146
Eucharistic Table 120
Example by living 131, 132
Faith 66, 68, 105
Fall of Jerusalem 9
Father, Heavenly 43, 63
Faithful 16, 104
Fire, Baptism of 41
Figs Fw. 159
Fiber in food 116, 117
Fermentation 116, 117, 122
Feathers 117
Ferocious beasts attack 97
Fasting 35, 63, 66, 106, 124
Flowers 120, 126, 149
First Christians 181
First Principles 189
Flaming Swords 41, 127
Flesh food 93, 102, 100, 184
Food, baked, boiled, frozen burnt, soaked Fw., 109
Food, peels, skins 119
Forbidden food 95
Forced Discipline 133
Fornication 62, 75
Fount of Living Water 40
Fruits 94, 102, 187
Frugal 126
Furs, leather, etc. 98
Gambling 132
Garment (white) 43, 101
Gases 55
Genetic Memory 100, 133
Genealogies 86
Genesis I, correct 94
Gifts, Divine 46
Gita Fw., 178
Gluttony 122, 126
Gnosis 47
Gnostic Christians 50, 123, 158

God is,
Harmony-Peace-Love 121
God Presence 36, 39
God Spelle 89, 188
GOLDEN TEXT OF
THE HOLY GRAIL 107, 151
Good 168
Good Samaritan 5, 71, 76, 132
Gospel origins 88, 173, 189
of Matthew 32, 189
of Mark John 189
of Luke 33
of John 188
Guides 132
Gymnosophists 96, 158/60, 178
Hadrian's time (John lives) 125
Hair 129
Harnack 161
Hate 13
Healer, Internal 67
Healing 18, 55, 66-68, 126/7
Healing Clergy 70, 71
Heart 74, 121, 128
Heavenly Hierarchy 63, 96, 131
Helen 29
Hermon 56
Herod, foster brother of,
Manaen (Gnostic John) 119
Herodotus 95
High, exalt or crucify 24
Hippocrates 73
Hitler 95
Holy Grail 151
Hook worm 79
Horses 109
How to eat 126
Hunger 120/1
Huxley 188
Hygienic cells 72
Hyperboreans 78, 95
Ignorance 60, 151

Illness, chronic 17
Illumination Fw., 89
Immanent Justice 93
Immortal Divine Spirit, Significance of Christ, a cross 158/160
Immunity Fw. 72, 73
India 156, 158
Infantile mind 98, 99
Initiates, Higher 145, 156
Initiations 60, 131, 150, 156, 188
Initiation, Johan(n)ine 51, 96, 97, 113, 114
Inherent Savior 71, 126, 127
Inner Anointing 119
Inner Healer, Healing 71, 127
Inner Ordinance 143, 145, 146
International Samaritan, Order 4, 5
Intestinal ferment 117
Irenaeus 25, 158, 183
Jacob's Ladder 99
James 160
Jehova 7, 97
Jerome 78, 85, 89
Jerusalem 7, 9, 171, 172
Jesus 85, 158, 180
Jews 8, 97, 150, 161
JOHN, BAPTIST (illumined), Fw., 8, 9, 10, 11, 28, 30, 31, 33 40, 50, 107, 171, 172, 176, 177
John Book 32, 87, 89
Jonas, Hans 49, 50, 53
Jordan Initiation 54, 56, 159
Josephus 158, 168, 169
Judas Zealot 165, 177
Juices 95, 120, 126
Karma 6, 25, 28, 62, 82, 93, 158
Keys to Heaven 106
Kill, Thou shalt not 93, 99
Kingdoms 92, 157
Koran 118, 158

Kristna Fw., 161, 178
Kukurepa 140, 141
Kundalini Chakras 56, 158
Kut Humi, Lal Singh 147
Latin vulgate 86
Lawless 125
Law of Love 45, 46
Laws of Life 22
Laws of Nature 13, 18
Levi 9
Life 109, 133
Light 43, 50
Library of Congress, first, Gospel (128 AD) 88
Library of Vatican 77
Limes, lemons 126
Lion 147
Lipsius 181
Living food Fw., 15, 18, 39, 106, 108
Living to eat 122, 126
Living Water 10, 18, 37, 40, 119, 123, 126-131
Living Word 26, 47, 119, 124
Longevity Fw., 144, 190
Lord 25, 38, 40
Love 44, 45, 92
Lubricant, digestive 116
Luminous Savior 52-54
Lung capacity 125
Maha Maitreyana Mandala 147
Maitreya 147, 149, 150
Manaen-Manaendros 119, 166
Manda 50 Mandaeans 31, 182
Mani 50, 156, 162
Marpa 140, 141, 142
Marcion (Marc John) 33, 88, 161
Manna 111
Mass, Holy 114, 120
Masturbate 107
Mastication 115

Mary Fw., 24, 31, 159
Mastery of Life 56
Matter, Material man 101
Meals, number per day 126
Mediums 105
Memory, Nature's 63, 84, 100
Menstruation 53, 93
Medicines 69, 72
Messengers 67, 82, 101
Messenger cells 70
Messiah 28, 152, 163
Milarepa Fw., 140
Military conflict 94
Mind dulling 101
Millenniums slumber 103
Milk 81, 82, 83, 94, 109
Merciful 25
Merinthus 119, 166, 183
Mixing food 121
Monophysites 4, 86, 87
Moses 8, 97, 98
Mother Nature 13, 41, 109
Murder 95
Mussolini 95
Matthias 33, 185
Nass-Aryans 34, 180
Nazarenes 87
Nature, Mother 12, 104, 109
Nebuchadnezzar 104
Needs, Lord knows our 57, 68
Nerves 70
Nestor 86
Never sick 60
Newman, J.H. 97
New Race 189, 190
Nivihim 156, 157
Ogdoad 149
Old English Bible 89
Old Latin Bible 89
One kind of food 121
Organs 74, 75

Original Scrolls 1
Order 75
Overcome self 34
Oxen 109
Papal Infallibility 97
Parables 60
Paradise 91, 95,
Paralysis 76
Patriarchate of Antioch 86
Paul 30
Paul and Peter quarrel 171
Peter 28, 31, 159
Peel 117, 119
Persia 156
Pesticides 95, 128, 129
Poison 128
Polycarp 183
Pots (not leper) Fw. 159
Pollution 129
Population excesses 95
Powers 130 of Yoga 180
Powers of Angels 67, 80, 82
Physician-Priests 131
Physiology 74
Plantain 128
Prayer 35, 63, 66, 68
Primal Man 51
Prodigal son 57-59
Prologue, Samaritan 1
Prophets 156
Protevangelion 11, 24, 160
Psychological nature 93, 94
Puma 147
Punishment 132
Punctuation, none in Bible 78
Purification 101, 102
Purification, intestinal 116, 117
Pyramids 111
Quarrel, Peter and Paul 30, 171
Qumran 53
Races 92

Rajneesh 143
Realms 101, 130
Red Lama 149
Reed, Violet Blossom 150
Reformatories 133
Regeneration 3, 56, 61, 132
Reincarnation 77, 162
Rejoicing 120, 121
Religion,
root meaning of Yoga 179
Reproductive fluids 107
Resurrection of Alexander 29
Resurrection of Jesus 85, 86
Resurrection of John 25, 158, 177
Resurrection of Simon 29
Revelations of John 183
Ripened fruit and clabber 116
Robes (white) 101
Rose 163, 165
Rosicrucian 166
Sacrifice 6, 7
Saints, all Christians 123
Saint of the Andes 189
Salad vegetables 94
Saliva 115
Salvation (Healed) 66, 151
Samariter 147
Samaritans 3, 28, 94
Sanctuary, Esoteric 146, 147
Satan 34, 41, 79, 80
Savior 48, 87, 158, 159
Seances 105, 106
School of Experience 133
Seed Foods 95
Self Healing Process 73
Self Mastery 130
Seminal losses 53, 145
Serpent 180
Seth, Elder 53
Sethians 53

Seventh day 130
Seven years in 7 days 62, 83
Sexual abuse 107
Sexual Interchange 145
Sexual passions 34
Sexual Purity 34, 135
Shambhala 52, 149
Simon Fw., 28, 103, 107, 159, 172, 178
Single Gospel 89, 160
Sins 42, 60
Skin Sores 67, 72
Slaughter 94
Slavemaster 58
Sleep 130
Slotosch, Martin 147
Slumber, Mankind 100, 103
Smell, altered 94
Snacking always 126
Snake bite 65
Sodom 53
Soil 16
Solitude 35
Solomon 154
Son of God 180
Son of man 24
Soul 61
Spelle, God 89
Spheres of Light 56
Spirit 3, 10, 14, 84, 128
Spiritualized man 46
Spiritualizing Dietetics 103, 123
Spontaneity 104, 119
Spring water 125
Stairway 99
Steinmann, Jean 30, 31
Stone Tablets, Moses 99
Sublimation 54, 153, 173
Suicide 154
Sun cooked (dead) food 112
Sunlight, Angel of 41

Superconsciousness 104, 129
Sweet fruits, excess 127
Szekely 4, 87, 94, 180
Table, Holy 118
Tatian 153
Therapeuts 96, 166
Temple Slaughterhouse 7, 9
Thanks to God 66, 83
Theodas, Theudas 170, 179
Think, so we become as 147
Tobacco 75
Toxic 118
Trajan, John Alive to 116
Transfiguration 49, 56
Translation by Mogner 139
Tray, earthenware 110
Tumors 67
Turkistan 52, 95, 148
Ulcers 67, 72
Unfoldment 155
Universal Religion 50, 154
University 43, 154
Vajrayana 134
Valentinus 32, 179
Vegetables 94, 102, 104, 110
Vetus Italica Fw., 89, 153
Vices 20
Virgin Birth 170, 178, 186
Vision 43
Vita Contemplativa 97
Vitalogical Sciences 73, 74, 138
Vital Life Fluid 105
Vitamins 111
Vitarian Diet 122
Voice 14, 15
Vulgate Latin 86
Water, Dead distilled 125
Water, Living 10, 18, 37
Water, Power, Angel of 36
Wastes, Cellular 67
Wastes, Intestinal 38

Wax, food coverings 116, 129
Wealth, exploiting disease 76
Weapons, Spiritual 35, 106
Weight excesses 102, 124
Wheat 112
White Friars Fw., 96
Wilderness, Voice Crying 14
Wise Men 156, 157
Word of God 14, 47, 149, 182
Words 99 Sacred 89-90
Work 130
Worry 120
Writings, Gnostic 53, 176, 182
Yahweh 8, 97
Yoga 178, 179, 180
Yoke 163, 179
Yohanan (see John)
You are what you eat 125
Zachary (Zacharius) Fw., 11, 24, 160, 167
Zebedee Fw., 161, 166
Zoroaster 51, 162

****

(We used Fw. as the abbreviation for the word "FOREWORD" which comes before page 1.)

The Healing God Spell of Saint John has been given Complete in 42 Chapters. (Plus 3 additional Chapters translated from the Spanish version, that were not originally translated) The Essene Gospel of John had 33.

+++

"When you invoke the Eternal," the Illumined replied, "Do not perform your devotion publicly. Exhibiting piety before others will get you no results from the Heavenly Self. When you pray, enter your Secret Chamber, within, close your mind to everything and meditate upon your Heavenly Self who dwells within the Inner Sanctuary, and your Holy Guardian who sees every secret act will reveal to you the Splendorous Self."

Made in the USA
Columbia, SC
23 February 2025